A PRACTICAL PSYCHOANALYTIC GUIDE TO REFLEXIVE RESEARCH

The Reverie Research Method

Joshua Holmes

Routledge
Taylor & Francis Group
LONDON AND NEW YORK

First published 2019
by Routledge
2 Park Square, Milton Park, Abingdon, Oxon OX14 4RN

and by Routledge
711 Third Avenue, New York, NY 10017

Routledge is an imprint of the Taylor & Francis Group, an informa business

British Library Cataloguing in Publication Data
A catalogue record for this book is available from the British Library

Library of Congress Cataloging in Publication Data
Names: Holmes, Joshua, 1983– author.
Title: A practical psychoanalytic guide to reflexive research : the reverie research method / Joshua Holmes.
Description: Abingdon, Oxon ; New York, NY : Routledge, 2018. |
Includes bibliographical references and index.
Identifiers: LCCN 2018014831 (print) | LCCN 2018020271 (ebook) |
ISBN 9780429467363 (Master) | ISBN 9780429884412 (Web PDF) |
ISBN 9780429884405 (ePub) | ISBN 9780429884399 (Mobipocket/Kindle) |
ISBN 9781138607026 (hardback) | ISBN 9781138607040 (pbk.)
Subjects: LCSH: Psychology–Research–Methodology. |
Qualitative research–Methodology. | Qualitative research–Psychological aspects. |
Psychoanalysis–Research–Methodology.
Classification: LCC BF76.5 (ebook) | LCC BF76.5 .H654 2018 (print) |
DDC 150.72/4–dc23
LC record available at https://lccn.loc.gov/2018014831

ISBN: 978-1-138-60702-6 (hbk)
ISBN: 978-1-138-60704-0 (pbk)
ISBN: 978-0-429-46736-3 (ebk)

Typeset in Bembo
by Out of House Publishing

For Ilya and Alkisti

CONTENTS

ACKNOWLEDGEMENTS

I thank Bob Hinshelwood and Nick Midgley for their generous and insightful supervision and for encouraging and challenging my research explorations during the PhD project which this book is a development of. For further encouragement and critical feedback, I also thank: Flavia Ansaldo, Evrinomy Avdi, Aaron Balick, Giovanni Colacicchi, Virge Eatough, Sue Kegerreis, Thomas Ogden, Sally O'Keeffe, Alejandra Perez, Mike Roper, Emily Stapley and Mary Target. I thank my psychoanalyst, who supported me as I worked on this book.

I thank my friends and family, for their love and support, especially my wife Alkisti, my sons Ilya and Alexander and my parents Ros and Jeremy.

I thank Sage publications for allowing me to present extracts from the following articles in this book:

Holmes, J. 'A comparison of clinical psychoanalysis and research interviews', *Human Relations* (66, 9) pp. 1183–1199. Copyright © 2013 Joshua Holmes. Reprinted by permission of Sage Publications. https://doi.org/10.1177/0018726712465315

Holmes, J. 'Countertransference in qualitative research: a critical appraisal', *Qualitative Research* (14, 2) pp. 166–183. Copyright © 2014 Joshua Holmes. Reprinted by permission of Sage Publications. https://doi.org/10.1177/1468794112468473

Holmes, J. 'Countertransference before Heimann: An historical exploration', *Journal of the American Psychoanalytic Association* (62, 4) pp. 603–629. Copyright ©2014 Joshua Holmes. Reprinted by permission of Sage Publications. https://doi.org/10.1177/0003065114546164

I thank Taylor & Francis, LLC and the *International Journal of Psycho-Analysis* for permitting me to reprint a substantial part of the following article in chapter 9 of this volume:

Holmes, J. 'Reverie-informed research interviewing', *International Journal of Psycho-Analysis* (98, 3) pp. 709–728. Copyright © 2017 Institute of Psychoanalysis, reprinted by permission of Taylor & Francis Ltd, www.tandfonline.com on behalf of Institute of Psychoanalysis.

This work was supported by the Economic and Social Research Council [grant number ES/J500045/1].

1

INTRODUCTION AND OVERVIEW

'Not sure ...' *Karl seems to drift into some sort of reverie. He sits upright with his sportsman's shoulders. Only traces of boyhood remain – a young, beardless face – but with intense weary eyes. He's glancing up to the left – searching inside, I think. And I wait, watching, sure enough that something will come out of the silence. He speaks quietly, bleakly, deeply.*

I sense my own keenness – willing more from Karl, tuning into the words. He speaks in a rather detached way about the difference between his depression and sadness. Sadness 'was' *(using the past tense)* 'the opposite of happy but depression'... *he pauses.* 'I dunno' – *another pause* ... 'just sort of ...' *the tone conveys movement – he will know soon – (I picture an empty glass about to be moved towards and filled from running water). And now stumbling towards a close-enough fit:* 'it's like it goes over all your feeling as a whole thing'. *With my own inward glance, I now imagine a field which snow has blanketed – 'gone over' it. I see stillness, and hear silence.* 'And it sort of governs your thoughts as well.' *Now I find myself wondering if an authoritarian figure has made Karl's bed (put the blanket in place). A few seconds of quiet, beholding the snowscape, before we are aware of it.* 'I'm imagining a blanket covering everything,' *I say. With the word* 'blanket' *Karl has said* 'yeah', *then he rests, and dismisses further exploration for the moment:* 'that's some incre-good example'.

I wrote this from my recollections of sitting in a room, for about an hour, with a 17-year-old young man.[1] We were involved in a 'research interview'. The recollection draws on intersubjective psychoanalytic theory which suggests that a two-person interaction entails a 'mutual meaning-making process' (Aron, 1992, p. 475), and that 'the analyst's associations to the patient's dreams are no less important than the patient's associations' (Ogden, 2001, p. 12). My own impressions, observations and reveries interact with Karl's responses to generate mutual and confirmatory understanding: '*that's some incre-good example*'.

What is a reverie approach to interviews?

Why do I start with this example? I want to show how in response to research interviews, the researcher's emotions, imagination and meaning-making capacities are activated, and how these processes can be put to good research use, rather than discarded as interference. The essence of this book and of the Reverie Research Method (RRM) is to show how, in response to qualitative research processes, researchers may foster a state of receptivity to emotional experience in which he or she may experience imagistic responses ('reveries'), which may then be linked to research data in order to better understanding the participant.

Understanding the 'inter view' (Kvale & Brinkmann, 2008) from a reverie perspective means studying the meeting of two minds – a collision of unconsciousness and consciousnesses – in such a way that the unconscious component can be thought about. Reverie-inspired mutual meaning-making involves a radical revision of what it means to be 'participant-centred' (Riach, 2009, p. 356). From this perspective, researcher neutrality becomes undesirable – and impossible in any case. A reverie approach to research interviews means the researcher learns to work with reference to *his or her own subjective responses*. This book aims to show how this can be done sensitively and systematically.

Reverie researching: who cares?

My focus is reverie-informed research and its consequences, potentialities and pitfalls. The book is aimed at two main constituencies: qualitative researchers interested in what psychoanalysis has to offer to their work, and psychoanalytic clinicians wanting to undertake psychoanalytically relevant research. The RRM may generate discussion and cross-fertilisation between them and point the way to new methodologies.

For qualitative researchers, a key question may be: 'Why, given its technical complexity and methodological problematics, is it so important to look inwardly ("practice reflexively"), and what can psychoanalysis add to this endeavour?' Some qualitative researchers have already made inroads towards interweaving psychoanalytic approaches into research methodologies (Devereux, 1967; Hunt, 1989; Hollway & Jefferson, 2013). Building on, although to some extent critical of this, the psychoanalytically inspired RRM offers a novel approach to reflexivity, reverie and intersubjectivity, showing how these can enhance the everyday qualitative methods of the research interview.

For psychoanalytic clinicians, a key question is: 'Is a research method possible that stays true to clinical realities?' (Holmes, 2017). Psychoanalysts, under external pressure to form an 'evidence base', but struggling with positivist notions of research, which are generally wholly remote from consulting room realities, may find themselves daunted, turned off and possibly irritated by demands which seem to fundamentally misunderstand the discipline (Chiesa, 2010). My hope is that this book may inspire clinicians to research and that clinicians may, via reverie-inspired methodology, find here a way of framing and conducting valid research, which at the same time prioritises unconscious processes and offers an ethical and close-up view of the human subject.

Comparing clinical psychoanalysis and research interviews

The significance of reverie, a complex and somewhat mythical concept, will emerge in the course of this book. But let's start with definitions. The Oxford English Dictionary defines reverie as 'being lost in thought', elegantly capturing the non-ego aspect and inwardness of reverie. Bion's technical elaboration of this, to be expounded later, led to his emphasis on 'mother's capacity for reverie' as descriptive of the state of mind which facilitates 'alpha function' (Bion 1962a, p. 307) – the way in which she receives, processes and returns, in manageable form, her infant's chaotic psychic experience.

As we shall see, the role of reverie in psychoanalysis was already present in Freud's early thinking, although more fully developed and theorised by Bion. Currently, the psychoanalyst Thomas Ogden, along with Antonio Ferro, are probably the foremost clinical proponents of the importance of reverie, especially when seen relationally. Ogden emphasises how reverie is a part of what it means to be alive as a 'human being' (e.g. Ogden 1994, p. 16; 1995, p. 696; 1997a, p. 6; 2001, p. 9). In doing so he reminds us that reverie is not limited to the clinic but underpins creativity. Reverie is an unforced, 'natural phenomenon'; and it is no less available and applicable in one-off encounters (which research interviews usually are) than in long-term ones. As Ogden (1992, p. 226) puts it: 'there is no difference in the analytic process in the first meeting and the analytic process in any other meeting'. Nevertheless, even if not limited to that location, the consulting room is certainly a good place to explore it. Aspects of psychoanalytic technique – attending to dreams and daydreams, free association, reflection, respecting silence, introspection – all are integral to reverie.

I shall show how these clinical principles can be reconsidered, reconfigured and applied in research methodology. Given that the research interview is a two-person dialogue, it is a good potential arena for mutually created meaning-making, and thus also a promising location for the exploration and application of reverie.

Three core concepts

Before exploring the practicalities of the RRM, three wider and interlinked themes will need to be considered: the nature of daydreaming (reverie); the search for understanding (research); and what it means to converse (interviewing).

Daydreaming

Reverie cannot be understood without reference to dreaming; etymologically the words are linked: 'rêve' is French for 'dream'. In 'knowing about' (Bion, 1965 p. 149) reverie, I have attempted – where possible – 'to be' *in* reverie and – *from* and *through* reverie – to research and write. My starting point is the view that reverie is not an intrinsically isolated and isolating phenomenon – although at times it can be – but to see it as relational. I justify this on two counts. First, as in my opening example, reverie is stimulated by the juxtaposition of two or more people's inner worlds. Second, even though one dreams alone, dreaming dissolves the ego, and therefore draws in an 'other' with which or whom the ego is in dialogue. A dream is a story about something distinct from one's conscious self; one that can be told to an 'other' – even if that other happens to be oneself! Reverie, and with it creativity, comes from a dawning awareness, from the 'edge of consciousness' (Waddell, 1984, p. 82).

Psychoanalytic discussions of reverie start from Bion (1962a, 1962b). Although before Bion the term reverie occasionally appears in the psychoanalytic literature, it refers in a non-technical sense to self-absorbed daydreaming. For example, Freud, in *The Interpretation of Dreams* (1900, p. 401) describes a mother in whom:

> ... thinking of the boy going into the water induced a reverie ['eine traumerei'] in which she saw herself taking him out of the water.

Just as Freud took the everyday term 'unconscious' and developed it into one of psychoanalysis's foundation stones, so Bion moved from the vernacular to develop a specialised psychoanalytic concept of reverie, although he deliberately avoids too much precision:

> I discuss the background of *emotional experience* from which it [the theory of reverie] has been abstracted. I shall do this in general terms without attempting scientific rigour.
>
> *Bion (1962a, p. 306; emphasis added)*

For Bion, the prototype of reverie is the feeding infant-and-mother. He sees reverie in terms of the mother's transformation of the baby's inchoate feelings into thoughts and meanings: 'the mother's capacity for reverie is the receptor organ for the infant's harvest of self-sensation gained by its conscious' (Bion, 1962a, p. 308). He links this with his 'theory of thinking' in which 'beta elements' (i.e. sensations) are transformed through this reverie process, via 'alpha function', into 'alpha elements' (i.e. thoughts).

Bion was influenced by Melanie Klein, although Klein herself appears not to have used the term 'reverie' ('Psychoanalytic Electronic Publishing-web' search). Bion links 'failures of alpha function', and therefore the incapacity for thinking which psychoanalysis aims to reverse, with the Kleinian notion of 'excessive projective identification'. This is a one-way process in which the infant expels overwhelming feelings such as rage and envy into the attendant object, i.e. the mother's breast. Bion's contribution, later developed and modified by Ogden, was the notion of 'realistic projective identification' (1962a,

p. 309), a to-and-fro movement of the minds' contents from baby to mother and back again. In Bion's hands, Klein's unidirectional projective identification becomes relational.

Bion's theory of reverie implies a number of other theoretical ingredients. First is *container/contained*. The mother's mind, figuratively, in Kleinian terms 'the breast', is the container into which the infant's sensations are projected. Second, if they can be contained, and not ignored or expelled by a mother in a state of intolerance of 'frustration', they become available for thinking, and, third, therefore, for 'communication'. I shall try to show how all three are relevant to researchers, for whom 'communication' encompasses not just verbal conversation but also publication.

In contrast to Bion's relational model, reverie in isolation is by definition incommunicable. Like maternal reverie, reverie-enriched researching involves balancing 'the free play of association' with 'logical scrutiny' (Ferenczi, 1950 [1919], p. 189). Devoid of reverie, research may verge into cold science, the 'mechanical brain' (Heimann, 1950, p. 82). But at the other extreme, reverie experience untempered by logical scrutiny, lies incomprehensibility.

Reverie can open alternative avenues into research data, and my aim here is to show how to apply reverie in research. Reverie-influenced researching becomes a *capacity* which may potentially be developed through practice and supervision. Reverie may be useful in overcoming blocks in research interviews, freeing moments of inarticulacy, or conversely enhancing emotional awareness when words block feelings. A second use of reverie lies in analysing interview transcripts. This has a more clearly defined *methodology* and, as I shall show, can be thought about systematically and in a group context.

When studying research interview transcripts, the 'free play of association' versus 'logical scrutiny', a toing-and-froing analogous to mother–baby interplay, involves sculpting understanding in relation to an experience of reverie, as it is worked and reworked. The writer has time for contemplation, and recruiting colleagues' perspectives, before committing finger to keyboard. In-the-moment 'live' reverie sharing, as in the case of Karl, involves greater risk. In that instance, I felt confident enough that what I said would contribute to the atmosphere of exploration. But – as we shall see – deciding how and whether to give voice to reverie is far from straightforward. There is always a tension between risk and security which reverie-influenced qualitative research entails.

What allows for the 'free play of association'/'logical scrutiny' process in the first place? When 'dreaming' cannot be separated from 'perceiving' (Ogden, 2003, p. 17) reverie cannot be distinguished from reality – that way lies delusion. Most people are fairly at home with benign daydreams of happiness, pleasure or success. But interviewing people who are suffering can induce disturbing fantasies or escape dreams in the interviewer. The excitement of 'awayness' (Sperling, 1953, p. 464) in reverie evokes and interacts with the counter-impulse towards safety and the fear of psychic freedom (cf. Fromm, 2001).

Researcher subjectivity and the interpersonal approach

Especially in psychological research, 're-search is me-search': 'behind the theory, method, analysis, ontology, epistemology, and methodology of qualitative research stands the personal biography of the researcher' (Denzin & Lincoln, 2000, p. 18). The same is true for the consenting participant. There is a balance to be struck between the wish to know and the reality that self-knowledge is elusive and potentially disruptive. 'At the centre of each person is an incommunicado element ... and this is sacred and most worthy of preservation' (Winnicott, 1965a, p. 187).

A brief discussion is needed here about three overlapping but distinct terms which I shall be using throughout: the *interpersonal*, *intersubjective* and *relational*. The term 'interpersonal' is typically associated with the American psychoanalyst and psychiatrist Harry Stack Sullivan (1954), founder of the William Alanson White clinic in Maryland. Sullivan was influenced by Sandor Ferenczi, and wanted to develop a psychiatry which valued connectedness and relationship as the key to psychic health and happiness; he criticised the aloof neutrality of the quasi-surgical analyst figure. Sullivan's collaborators included Harold Searles and Freida Fromm-Reichman, both pioneers of psychoanalytic work with psychotic patients, and also Erich Fromm. Fromm (2001), a refugee from Nazi Germany, developed his own existential-ethical approach to psychoanalysis which emphasised freedom, relatedness and the overcoming of 'existential angst'.

The concept of intersubjectivity in psychoanalysis has been systematically developed by Stolorow & Atwood (2002). They contest the 'myth of the isolated mind' (*ibid.*, p. 203) and, drawing on field theory, suggest that all human experience, including thinking itself, should be seen as entailing the interpenetration of subjectivities. Their work draws on Daniel Stern's (1985) empirical studies of parent–child communication, which describe and theorise patterns of attunement and mis-attunement, especially in the pre-verbal first year of life. A second major influence on the intersubjectivists is the work of Donald Winnicott. Like Klein, the term reverie does not appear to have been used by Winnicott, but the concept Bion describes is implicit in Winnicott's view of a mother's intuitive understanding of and response to her infant's needs. Winnicott's intersubjectivism is illustrated by his model of everyday creativity in which the infant's hallucinatory longing for the breast is intuitively responded to by the mother in a such a way that the breast appears 'as though by magic', just when the child wants and imagines (or 'image'-ines – I shall show later how the RRM has at its core visual imagery). For Winnicott, this illusion of having conjured the desired object into experience is the basis for healthy omnipotence and the germ of the transitional space, a creative buffer zone between desire and reality.

The third term is the adjective 'relational'. In using it I am picking a somewhat eclectic pathway through a number of psychoanalytic thinkers including Freud himself, Ferenczi, Fromm, Bion, Winnicott and the contemporary psychoanalysts Ogden and Ferro. However, although sympathetic to the relational viewpoint, I do not necessarily subscribe to Relational Psychoanalysis as a 'movement' (see Mitchell

1990; Aron 1995; Benjamin 2004). But the founding principles of relationality – that a psychoanalytic relationship entails the meeting of two unconsciousnesses, which together create a mutual 'third' – is one that has been a profound influence, and which I argue can be partially transposed from the therapeutic into the research setting. The term relational is also included in the title of the British 'Object Relations' school, starting with the work of Melanie Klein and Ronald Fairbairn. The view underpinning this book is that 'object relations', in the sense of unconscious relational dispositions, play a central part in qualitative research interviewing, and can thus be put to empirical use.

In line with this range of conceptualisations of the relational, the search for self-knowledge, while requiring a degree of one-person introspection (including being 'at home' with silence), is, I argue, essentially interpersonal.

If we consider subjective experience accessed through reverie as potentially emanating from the intersubjectivity of researcher and participant, it becomes imperative to find ways to communicate '*from*' reverie but (possibly in contrast to the self-revelation in Relational Psychoanalysis) 'not often … directly about' (Ogden, 1997b, p. 568) the researcher's inner world. The researcher needs to find ways to 'use' his or her reverie in the service of greater understanding of the participant, without imposing an experience upon the participant.

This prompts further terminological distinctions. Bion's theory of reverie formed part of the new ways of understanding countertransference. This is no longer a technical term for the analyst's neuroses from which, via 'training analysis' and supervision, she or he is 'cured', thereby clearing the deck for uncontaminated patient-focused interpretation. In the contemporary model, by analogy with mother and infant, the analyst contains the patient's projections, subjects them to his/her alpha function, whereupon they are converted into word-based thoughts, and therapeutically communicated and so 'returned' to the patient.

Countertransference and research conversations

Along these lines, Paula Heimann's (1950) classic paper, 'On counter-transference', discussed in the next chapter, argues that the analyst's countertransference is a useful tool in understanding patients' feelings and dispositions. Bion's 'reverie' is the container – a receptive, free-associating, musing, empathic state of mind. The 'contained' are the unnamed feelings waiting to be named and re-introjected once the analyst's alpha function gets to work on them. Here countertransference is an aspect of reverie. With the help of Ogden (1992), I term this process 'relational reverie'. This goes beyond countertransference seen in terms of projective identification. It suggests that analyst and patient together generate a 'third' arising from the combined unconscious processes of both parties. The analyst's responses evoked by the patient's projections are a product neither of his/her own neuroses (Freud's original position), nor a more – or less – accurate reflection of the patient's (the Heimann model), but a novel co-creation that 'belongs' to neither alone. I shall argue that this model can be applied to research interviews in order to generate new and useful research hypotheses.

Chapter outlines

Chapter 2 is a critical exploration of how psychoanalysts have understood and made use of their own subjectivity as a clinical tool. Freud, from studying his public papers, and private letters, appeared to feel both intrigued and disturbed by the topic. I offer a 'qualitative analysis', in the sense of an archival investigation, of these writings, including early letters on the subject to Jung, Ferenczi and others. Chapter 3 moves on to later developments – already touched on above – including an account of the evolution of the concepts of 'countertransference' and 'projective identification'. The final section of the chapter addresses the contemporary uses of reverie, including related concepts such as 'negative capability' and 'containment'.

Chapter 4 moves from psychoanalytic practice and theory into the research arena and makes the case for reverie-informed strategies in relation to research interviewing. How and why researchers have come to value and draw on psychoanalytic ideas and methods is scrutinised. In Chapter 5 the paradigms of reflexivity in research and therapeutic contexts are contrasted. The chapter frames the research interview as a coming together of human subjects. Chapter 6 looks at ethical aspects of qualitative research, arguing that ethical concerns – attempting to overcome the dehumanisation of the subject implicit in some traditional research methodology – override narrow research aims, but also that ethically minded research will produce fuller research findings.

Chapter 7 introduces some of the early data from which the RRM evolved, and a further rationale for their use is offered. This is followed in Chapter 8 by a specific focus on the work of the psychoanalyst Thomas Ogden, and how his approach to psychoanalysis has inspired elements of the thinking behind RRM.

Chapter 9 shows RRM in action. Through two examples of research interviews, I explore how reverie shaped the interview process. I look at reverie in relation to rapport-building, breaking impasse, gaining understanding and as a springboard for further research questions. I argue that researcher 'neutrality' is both an impossibility and runs counter to certain research aims.

Chapter 10 shows how the RRM can be applied to data analysis of interview transcripts. The process revealed how material 'housed' (Morgenroth, 2010) in such scripts may be accessed, and how this leads to new understandings of participant dialogues and participant–interviewer interactions.

Thus far my examples of RRM in action draw mainly on my own experiences conducting research interviews, and the reverie generated within these. Chapters 11 and 12 show the responses and outcomes of researchers to reverie teaching groups. The final chapter is a reprise of the theoretical and empirical aspects of the RRM, and discusses their implications for the two potential target audiences: psychoanalyst-researchers and qualitative researchers interested in augmenting reflexive approaches through drawing on psychoanalysis.

Terminology

I hope the reader of this book will develop his or her own understanding of the terms and concepts I draw on. However, in partial reassurance, Chapters 2 and 3 locate and discuss terms such as 'reverie', 'countertransference' and 'research interviewing', hoping to extend the meanings and reverberations they evoke.

Note

1 In the examples in this book, distinguishing details about participants have been disguised and participants consented to take part in the interviews and groups presented.

2

FREUD AND THE ROLE OF SUBJECTIVITY IN PSYCHOANALYSIS

Since Bion's (1962b, p. 36) description of 'mother's capacity for reverie', the term has been widely used in psychoanalytic writing. In keeping with Bion's deliberately chosen practice, however, rarely is it clearly defined or justified.

From a pre-psychoanalytic perspective, the Oxford English Dictionary charts the history of the word. For over four centuries it has been used in various ways to denote a state of joy; sexual lust; and a 'fantastical notion'. Here is an early example from Locke (1997 [1690], cited in the Oxford English Dictionary, 1997):

> ... when ideas float in our mind, without any reflection or regard of the understanding, it is that which the French call Revery; our language has scarce a name for it.

And later:

> Walking around in a sad reverie ... unconscious to the world around her.
>
> *Irving Sketch (1820, I.145, cited in Oxford English Dictionary, 1997)*

Psychoanalytic description of reverie before Bion

Before Bion, reverie was seen by psychoanalytic writers as equivalent to the vernacular notion of daydreaming. The 'Psychoanalytic Electronic Publishing-web' archive retrieves 78 articles containing the word 'reverie' predating Bion's (1962b) contribution (search conducted in January 2017). In this pre-Bion psychoanalytic literature, the word conveys the sense either of an all-consuming dream or, more usually, a daydream (Speziale-Bagliacca, 2008). Ellis (1919, p. 405) quotes a patient describing a daydream-within-a-dream:

> I dreamt I was sitting in front of a fire day-dreaming. The room was apparently a kind of salon, with French windows to the left. I seemed to be the only person in the room and I was wrapped in a reverie of most engrossing nature.

'Reverie' evokes the image of a daydreamer who 'loses' (e.g. Kempf, 1919, p. 45) her- or himself through 'lapsing' (Stern, 1948, p. 527), 'sinking' (Metman, 1957, p. 63) or 'falling into' (Dooley, 1930, p. 212; Swackhamer, 1937, p. 196; Deutsch, 1954, p. 296; Bergler, 1955, p. 169) something 'profound' (Tauber, 1949, p. 325). The words used to describe entering a reverie state are ones usually associated with falling asleep. However, reverie seems also to indicate engulfing ('wrapped', Ellis, 1919) introspection: '... he lived the life of a vagabond, going about unwashed and hungry, sleeping out of doors in winter weather and falling into long periods of reverie' (Swackhamer, 1937, p. 196).

Reverie in these examples denotes non-relatedness: an 'absence' or 'awayness' (Sperling, 1953, p. 464), sometimes likened to the moment between waking and sleeping (Murphy, 1958), trance-like states, in which the world is experienced as passing us by, until a word, a noise, a pat on the shoulder or some other stimulus snaps us out of it and we may only be retrospectively aware of having drifted off like this (this phrase 'drifting off' seems appropriate here, as it does of falling asleep, with its watery connotations).

From the outside, we may see a person in reverie as 'entranced'; their distractedness may be amusing or disturbing. If we ask them what was passing through their mind during these moments, often they say they 'can't remember', or 'nothing'. This 'forgetting' is associated with reverie and the need for privacy which makes up part of the healthy psyche (Winnicott, 1963). Accessing reverie states involves 'tampering with an essential inner sanctuary of privacy, and therefore with one of the cornerstones of our sanity' (Ogden, 1994, p. 12).

There are several early psychoanalytic attempts to theorise daydreaming. Montani & Pietranera (1946) and Enckell (1982) use the analogy of film to describe the unconscious: a 'language of images' (Montani & Pietranera, 1946, p. 179). To 'transmit imaginative thoughts' they must be translated into 'verbal judgments', which 'deforms' and 'unindividualizes' the original thought (*ibid.*, p. 180). The sense is that dream states, whether 'waking dreaming' as in reverie, or asleep, can never be fully transmitted to another through words.

For Freud there is no sharp dividing line between night and daydreams; they are 'analogous' (Freud, 1900, p. 491). Furthermore, daydreams

> stand in much the same relation to the childhood memories from which they are derived as do some of the Baroque palaces of Rome to the ancient ruins whose pavements and columns have provided the material for the more recent structures.
>
> ibid., *p. 492*

Freud's reverie here is child-like and non-communicative, but also potentially constructive. Kris (1946, p. 232) made a link between free association and the 'stream of consciousness novel', in which 'the preconscious reverie becomes the paramount way of expression' – a hint of the idea of *creative reverie* which Bion later developed.

By the 1920s, the importance of dreamlike waking states was gaining recognition in psychoanalysis. But at this stage reverie was viewed as essentially intrapsychic, originating in early 'primitive' childhood constellations. As we have mentioned and will elaborate below, Bion reconceptualised reverie as relational, i.e. emanating from the interpsychic realm, since events in the inner world are evoked and stimulated by those in the intimate interpersonal field. But before considering Bion's contribution and those of his successors, we need to look at how the *analyst's subjectivity* was conceptualised as psychoanalysis evolved – i.e. the theory and practice of countertransference.

Countertransference

Sandler, Holder & Dare (1970, p. 84) suggest that the 'counter' in countertransference could mean either: a) something going on in parallel to the patient's transferences (as in 'counterpart'),[1] or b) a reaction to them (as in 'counteract'). The prefix 'counter-' can indeed mean either 'against' or 'in return' (Oxford English Dictionary, 1997), as can the original German 'gegen' of 'gegenubertragung'.

To the extent to which countertransference was seen as a parallel process (i.e. sense (a) above), theorists were imputing transference reactions towards the patient on the part of the analyst, comparable to the patient's towards the analyst (Reich, 1951; Gitelson, 1952; Tower, 1956). The second implication, (b) of 'counter' leads to the idea of countertransference as reactive. Here countertransference is conceived as a response to the patient's transference. As Heimann (1977, p. 318) points out, had Freud wanted to refer to the analyst's 'own' transference he would have said so, rather than creating a new hybrid word, 'countertransference': instead 'the prefix "counter" characterizes the phenomenon as a specific response to the patient' (*ibid.*).

'Counter' works both ways. The patient's transference is also generated 'counter' to something – i.e. the presence of the analyst. Lacan (1951, cited in Etchegoyen, 1991, p. 267) argued that transference, 'located' in the patient, nevertheless includes the analyst's emotional response to the patient, made up of 'the sum of prejudices, passions, perplexities and … insufficient information on the part of the analyst at a given moment of the dialectic process'. Although he later moderated this view (Etchegoyen, 1991), it shows the importance Lacan placed on the subjective position of the analyst in relation to the patient, and how this is integral to the development of a transference relationship. We see here psychoanalytic thinkers struggling with ways to conceptualise how the interpersonal can emerge from the intrapsychic worlds of two interacting subjects.

Countertransference was a controversial and feared experience. Etchegoyen (1991, p. 267) takes a firm line:

> [The] constants of the setting ... and ... the analytic reserve ... justify our defining transference as that which comes from the patient and countertransference as the analyst's response, and not the other way around.

Freud on countertransference

But Freud's position was more nuanced than is usually recognised. He is usually portrayed as having little to say about countertransference, and when he did mention it, he was thought to have seen it as an impediment to analytic work:

> ... the narrow Freudian view of countertransference is that it interferes with the analytic work. In essence, Freud regarded it as the analyst's transference to the patient. The construct was not viewed as positive or useful until the arrival of Paula Heimann's (1950) classic paper in which she made clear for the first time that the analyst's reaction might actually be a useful clue to what was happening inside the patient.
>
> *Gabbard (2005, p. 185)*

This is a widely held view, but Freud – a voluminous correspondent – has much to say about countertransference in his letters (Freud, 1909, 1910a, 1910b, 1911, 1913, 1917a, 1917b, 1931; see Holmes, 2014). It did also get a public mention by Freud, albeit minimally, and more critically (Freud 1910c, 1912). This downplaying was, as we shall see, probably more 'political' than scientific.

Freud's first documented reference to 'countertransference' is in a letter to Jung in 1909, in response to Jung's confessed emotional and probable sexual entanglement with a patient. Freud dismissively responds:

> ... no lasting harm is done. They [the experiences to which Jung had 'confessed'] help us develop the thick skin we need to dominate "countertransference", which is after all a permanent problem for us; they teach us to displace our own affects to best advantage. They are a "*blessing in disguise*".
>
> *Freud (1909, pp. 230–231, emphasis in original)*

The word 'countertransference' is not elaborated, but Freud frames the analyst's unconscious responses to patient communications as a 'blessing in disguise' (Freud used the English phrase in a letter otherwise written in German), which, it implies should be 'displaced' and used, rather than eliminated. This resonates with Ogden's description, to which we shall return, of how intersubjective communication is experienced in reverie, but may be 'disguised' as a narcissistic- or irrelevant-seeming daydream: the therapeutic relevance of reverie is almost always a 'retrospective discovery' (Ogden, 1997c, p. 720).

Freud returned to the theme in his 1910 address at the opening of the Second Psycho-Analytical Congress in Nuremberg. Freud described the 'inexorable and exhausting' feelings absorbed by the analyst when 'the patient had to say everything himself' (1910c, p. 141). Seeing the treatment as 'made up of two parts' produced a 'more friendly air' (*ibid.*). The analyst's connection with his or her own emotional world made the analytic situation bearable. But this new perspective presents a problem: to the extent that countertransferential 'two-partedness' is acknowledged, Freud's valued analytic objectivity and detachment are under threat.

Freud conceded: 'a therapeutic procedure cannot be carried out in the same way as a theoretical investigation' (*ibid.*, p. 142). On psychoanalysis – 'new things' were being discovered every day, including 'important amplification' from analysts other than Freud himself (*ibid.*). Just as the analyst was no longer the sole arbiter of what goes on in the consulting room, so Freud here is acknowledging that he was no longer master of the analytic world, but could benefit from the contributions of his students and colleagues. His phrase 'made up of two parts' (*ibid.*, p. 141) could perhaps refer both to the analytic dyad and the analytic community.

The much-quoted passage continues:

> … the 'counter-transference' … arises in him [the analyst] as a result of the patient's influence on his unconscious feelings, and we are almost inclined to insist that he shall recognize this counter-transference in himself and overcome it … we have noticed that no psycho-analyst goes further than his own complexes and internal resistances permit.
>
> ibid., *pp. 144–145*

The analyst's own blind spots and neuroses block, restrict or channel his understanding of the patient's material. But Freud also implies that through deeper self-understanding comes a smoother analytic path. The standard reading of this is that analysts who are thoroughly analysed will be equipped to work well analytically because their countertransference feelings have been 'overcome' (Cole, 1922).

But Freud's comment could also be taken to mean that if the analyst is at home with his or her countertransference it can be used for the patient's benefit. Countertransference has to be 'recognised' as well as 'overcome'. Freud later says that when patients fall in love with analysts this signifies for the analyst 'a valuable piece of enlightenment and a useful warning against any tendency to a countertransference' (Freud, 1915, p. 160). Again, at face value this is merely saying 'watch out for your countertransference' – i.e. don't get emotionally involved – and 'don't fool yourself into thinking the patient is "really" in love with you'. But it could also imply 'your countertransference love or erotic interest can be "valuable" and an "enlightenment" about the patient's inner world'.

At this stage in the evolution of psychoanalysis, countertransference was seen as a potentially disruptive force needing to be reined in via the analyst's personal analysis and self-awareness. If the patient's love is 'transferential' (rather than 'real') then by the same token so too is the analyst's. Sexual feelings in the analyst are presented as a 'counter-response' to those in the patient. For Freud, the 'enlightenment' countertransference provides is 'valuable' in that it shows how the patient may conflate real love and transference love, and provides a warning for the analyst not to fall into the same trap. Freud's recognition of the importance of the spontaneous (*ibid.*, p. 162) emergence of patient feelings (in this example, transference-love), contrasts with his guarded, unspontaneous attitude to the analyst's countertransference, which must be 'overcome'.

This represents Freud's publicly expressed viewpoint. However, two years earlier, in a letter to Binswanger, he had put forward an alternative view on the analyst's spontaneity in relation to countertransference, suggesting that

> counter-transference ... is – technically – among the most intricate in psychoanalysis. Theoretically I believe it is much easier to solve. What we give to the patient should, however, be *a spontaneous affect*, but *measured out consciously* at all times, to a greater or lesser extent according to need. In certain circumstances a great deal, but never from one's own unconscious ... One must, therefore, always recognise one's counter-transference and overcome it, for not till then is one free oneself. *To give someone too little because one loves him too much is unfair to the patient and a technical error.* This is all far from easy, and perhaps one has to be older for it, too.
>
> *Freud (1913, p. 112, emphasis added)*

In 1913 Freud had yet to fully develop his tripartite id/ego/superego model of the mind, but nevertheless this passage could be understood in terms of the structural model. Feelings arise in the analyst; these could be countertranferential, representing the analyst's own id-driven needs (e.g. to be loved), so the superego might 'say': 'this is bad, hold back'. But these feelings also 'represent' a therapeutic response to the patient's need. So the more mature – less superego-dominated – ego might 'say': 'those feelings are partly representing your own need to be loved, but also the patient's need for love, so don't throw the baby out with the bathwater – be appropriately warm'. This moves in the direction of a model in which patient's need for love, analyst's need for love, and their need to give love correlate and can be used for the former's benefit. The analyst's 'thinking mind' appraises this and meets out the ethically and therapeutic amount of love that the patient needs (in an ideal world!).

For the patient, Freud's 'fundamental rule' (Freud, 1925, p. 40) of free association was based on *un*measured spontaneity. In the Binswanger letter Freud acknowledges the potential value of carefully handled countertransference. Here we have a model in which feelings/affect/unconscious come up 'from below' in a spontaneous way; the ego/conscious-self/cognitive apparatus then appraises these and 'measures them out' rather than either blurting them out, 'wildly', or entirely denying or suppressing them as a harsh superego might demand. As in his 1909 letter to Jung, he suggests that through experience the analyst will do best to 'surmount' his countertransference. He develops the intriguing paradox of *measured spontaneity*, but this idea does not appear to have been developed much further by Freud himself.

Nevertheless, the analyst's 'capacity for spontaneity' (Ogden, 1995, p. 696) is central to contemporary discussions on the clinical application of countertransference. These can range from something akin to Freud's notion of measured spontaneity to a more unrestrained expression of feelings. After experiencing reverie: 'we ... attempt to speak ... from what we are *thinking about feeling*' (Ogden, 1997b, p. 568, emphasis added). By contrast, Birksted-Breen (2012, p. 828) describes a more spontaneous intervention which followed her experience of a 'powerful visual image'. The 'measured' part came in her actively attempting to 'regain' something unmeasured – an 'unfocused state of mind' (*ibid.*). An interpretation may be spoken and only later is it thought about.

Summarising Freud's views on countertransference, he held a somewhat contradictory picture of the analyst's subjectivity as both a positive and negative force in the analytic process. 'Countertransference' was first mentioned as a tactful suggestion that Jung needed more analysis in 1909. But Freud also suggested, if suitably 'dominated', that it could be used to the analyst's advantage. Next, in his 1910 and 1915 papers, Freud depicts countertransference as a serious obstacle to appropriate analytic responsiveness. Underlying both views is an awareness of analysis as a 'two person' process. Freud notes the interactive aspect: how the patient's material evokes countertransference reactions on the part of the analyst. Although Freud sensed that emotional detachment in the analyst was unhelpful, he never developed his idea that countertransference could be put to good use, other than through his 1913 coinage of 'spontaneous affect ... measured out consciously'.

This endorsement of carefully handled countertransference laid the bedrock for subsequent theories, but he never quite made this publicly known. Here he is in a letter to Jung:

> I believe an article on 'counter-transference' is sorely needed; *of course we could not publish it, we should have to circulate copies among ourselves.*
>
> *Freud (1911, p. 476, emphasis added)*

It seems likely that Freud decided that were he publicly to say that countertransference could be useful – that analysts have feelings too – it would threaten his image of the psychoanalyst as a detached surgeon of the soul, and might encourage 'wild analysis' (Freud, 1910c). But in private, Freud seemed aware that it was unavoidable that the analyst's unconscious feelings would be evoked in relation to the patient, and, moreover, from the therapeutic point of view this process could be beneficial to the analysis.

Ferenczi

Further development of these ideas came from Ferenczi, Freud's protégé and 17 years his junior, who developed an elaborate, and at the time unorthodox, theory of the usefulness of analytic subjectivity (Rachman, 1993). Ferenczi (1950 [1919], p. 189) wrote about *countertransference control*:

> ... only when ... [the analyst's] feelings towards the patient tend to overstep the right limits in either a positive or a negative sense, only then can the doctor "let himself go" during the treatment as psycho-analysis requires of him.

In contrast to Freud's 'measured spontaneity', Ferenczi here makes the paradoxical and uncomfortable suggestion that it is only when things get a bit out of hand that countertransference produces therapeutic benefit. Lest this be seen as a prescription for analytic acting out, Ferenczi continued:

> Analytic therapy ... requires of him [the analyst] the free play of association and phantasy, the full indulgence of *his own unconscious* ... only in this way is it possible to grasp intuitively the expressions of the *patient's unconscious* ... on the other hand, the doctor must subject the material ... to a logical scrutiny, and in his dealings and communications may only let himself be guided by the result of this mental effort.
>
> ibid. *(emphasis in original)*

Ferenczi is here advocating 'internal' licence, strictly coupled with 'logical scrutiny' and 'mental effort'. Ferenczi was aware that countertransference feelings would inevitably arise in the course of treatment, irrespective of how 'well analysed' the analyst was:

> ... even the analysed individual is not so independent of peculiarities of character and actual variations of mood as to render the supervision of the counter-transference superfluous.
>
> *Ferenczi (1950 [1919], p. 187)*

Where Freud had suggested self-analysis as a way of dealing with countertranference, Ferenczi appears to be the first advocate of the need for supervision, although whether this is, in Casement's (1985) terms 'internal' or external supervision is not clear. For him the aim is not to 'overcome' countertransference (Freud, 1913) but to facilitate its understanding and put it to good use. 'Overcoming' countertransference, in the sense of denying or repressing it, would be undesirable: the analyst's susceptibility to 'moods, sympathies and antipathies, as well as impulses' is precisely what allows him or her to understand the patient's psychic conflicts (Ferenczi, 1950 [1919], p. 186). But, ever aware of going too far towards untempered 'indulgence', Ferenczi argues that 'analysis demands of the physician, not only a firm control of his own narcissism, but also a sharp watch on his emotional reactions of every kind' (1955 [1928], p. 95).

Underpinning Ferenczi's vision of countertransference as inevitable and essential is his understanding of the analyst as a human subject. Ferenczi's humanity comes across in his acknowledgement of the analyst's feelings, transference/countertransference-driven mistake-making and honest presence. We see a conceptual progression here from countertransference, seen first as intrapsychic, towards viewing the analyst's inner world as resonating with that of the patient. We shall see how the RRM also requires a comparable combination when using reverie in research settings.

Ferenczi's views on analyst self-revelation are controversial. Ferenczi saw it as 'professional hypocrisy' (Ferenczi, 1955 [1928], p. 158) that analysts promise to listen to the patient's associations, but when some difficulty or unpleasant feeling arises, keep their own feelings under wraps. The solution is 'to make the source of the disturbance in us fully conscious and to discuss it with the patient' (*ibid.*, p. 159). This is a revolutionary and still contentious precept (Ehrenberg, 1995). Not only is Ferenczi saying that analysts must be in touch with their emotional responses, but that they must also find ways to share these feelings with the patient. For Ferenczi, a lack of openness about feelings can recreate for the patient childhood traumas of parental emotional withdrawal.

Today, the principle that the analyst must attend to her or his feelings and put them to therapeutic use would be widely accepted. The debate is about technique. Should countertransference reactions be *explicitly* 'shared' with the analysand (e.g. Ehrenberg, 1995, Renik, 2004), or transmuted into communications that do not necessarily refer directly to the analyst's feelings (e.g. Ogden, 1995)?

Openness, Ferenczi argues, is especially important in the face of mistakes: 'it would almost seem to be of advantage occasionally to commit blunders in order to admit afterwards the fault to the patient' (1955 [1928], p. 159). This attitude found its zenith in Ferenczi's 'mutual analysis' treatment of Elisabeth Severn, as describe in Ferenczi's (1932) clinical diary. During this treatment, Ferenczi confirms the patient's suspicions that he had been concealing hatred when he reveals to her that his dealings with her had stirred his own hatred for his mother. Later Ferenczi and Severn changed places as analyst and patient (literally – Ferenczi lay on the couch, something which Antonio Ferro also admits to having done with a patient – Ferro & Nicoli, 2017). Without endorsing role-reversal between patient and analyst, this foreshadowed the idea that mistakes in the analytic setting are inevitable and can be put to good use (e.g. Winnicott, 1956; Casement, 2002), and research which shows the therapeutic benefits of doing so (Safran & Muran, 2000).

For Ferenczi (1955 [1928], p. 160) confidence in the analyst's honesty 'establishes the contrast between the present and the unbearable traumatogenic past'. This parallels Winnicott's recognition of the importance of the analyst's awareness of hate as an essential step towards gaining trust: 'if the patient seeks objective or justified hate he must be able to reach it, else he cannot feel he can reach objective love' (1949, p. 72).

In summary, Ferenczi made strides in the theorisation of analytic subjectivity, and in showing how it might be therapeutically useful. He recognised that countertransference feelings are a universal feature of all analytic treatments, no matter how 'well-analysed' the analyst. He insisted that personal analysis and supervision were essential in learning to 'guide' (rather than overcome) the countertransference. For him, psychoanalysis is a living exploration of affective communication between two people. He suggests that analysts must be aware of the totality of their emotional responses, and must find creative ways of relating and relaying this to the patient. Without this honesty, spontaneity and control, analytic treatment will fail. The analyst must not be sterile and unresponsive. Ferenczi recognised this openness to feelings as a guarantor of the analyst's humanity, but also the importance of subjecting these feelings to 'logical scrutiny'.

Other early contributions

Other early psychoanalytic authors highlight the importance of the analyst's emotional connectedness. Ella Sharpe (1927) shows how there is a close relationship between the analyst's and the patient's transferences and later suggests that through personal analysis, countertransference is not eliminated; rather, the analyst 'will not be afraid to recognize in himself signs that betray impatience, anger, and embarrassment. He will note when he hesitates to give interpretations' (Sharpe 1947, p. 4).

Reik (1933, p. 327) writes of the analyst needing to find his or her bearings when in the midst of 'the chaos of the living psychic process' as opposed to thinking about 'analytic theory'; Strachey (1934, p. 150) advocates 'emotionally "immediate" interpretations'; Low (1935, p. 2) argues that 'emotional activity' is the route to 'correct interpretations'; Fenichel (1939, p. 184) champions 'humanness'; and Ferenczi's analysand Michael Balint viewed the analyst's 'personality' – and therefore, presumably, the capacity to be helpfully in touch with emotions – as being the most important factor in the shape of an analysis (Balint & Balint, 1939).

Paula Heimann

Heimann's (1950) paper opened a new chapter in thinking about countertransference (Hinshelwood, 2012), in that she foregrounds and endorses the relational aspects of the analyst–patient dyad. She opens her paper by asserting that *fear* of countertransference leads psychoanalysts to 'avoid any emotional response and to become completely unfeeling and "detached"' (Heimann, 1950, p. 81). She argues that the aim of personal therapy for analysts is not to 'turn him [sic – the analyst] into a mechanical brain which can produce interpretations on the basis of a purely intellectual procedure' (*ibid.*, p. 82). The analyst needs to be aware of his or her own feelings before making interpretations:

> ... in the comparison of feelings roused in himself with the patient's associations and behaviour, the analyst possesses a most valuable means of checking whether he has understood or failed to understand his patient.
>
> *Heimann (1950, p. 82)*

She suggests that the countertransference is the patient's 'creation' (*ibid.*, p. 83):

> the analyst's immediate emotional response to his patient is a significant pointer to the patient's unconscious processes and guides him towards fuller understanding.

Based on the Kleinian concept of 'projective identification' (see below) she views countertransference feelings as affects which start life in the patient. In her model, countertransference is a therapeutic tool guiding the analyst's thoughts towards the patient's 'most urgent' associations and is a 'useful criterion for the selection of interpretations' (*ibid.*).

Later, Heimann (1960), having now distanced herself from Melanie Klein (Tonnesmann, 1989), describes the *non*-therapeutic implications of countertransference – either its excessive use or its dismissal. The 'un-critical use of countertransference' refers to the use of feelings in the analyst without relating them to the 'actual data in the analytic situation' (Heimann, 1960, p. 153). Here countertransference becomes an 'excuse' for any emergent feeling, and perhaps acting out, in the analyst.

The other extreme, which according to Heimann is especially a problem among analytic 'candidates', is when, through a misunderstanding of Freud, analysts have 'endeavoured to become inhuman' and disconnected with their feelings (*ibid.*, p. 151). Here she returns to Freud's idea that extensive analysis will help the analyst dissect out his or her own neurosis from the patient's material: 'when the analyst in his own analysis has worked through his infantile conflicts and anxieties … he will not impute to his patient what belongs to himself' (1950, p. 83). If that can be discounted, she suggests, when unexpected feelings arise in a 'well-analysed' analyst, they must be emanating from the patient (i.e. through projective identification). This putative well-analysed analyst will be able to 'easily establish' what comes from the patient and what 'belongs to himself' (*ibid.*).

Heimann makes a distinction between 'interfering' and 'useful' countertransference. But as will be developed below, what is missing here is a perspective of mutual influence. While Heimann was clearly influenced by Bion, there is a significant difference: Bion's theory of maternal reverie is relational, and even more so as developed by Ogden, while Heimann's countertransference seems to 'belong' either to the analyst or to the patient.

Other Kleinian-inspired and British object relations perspectives

Several other theoretical advances were made in the 1950s. Racker (1953, p. 314) confronts the collective 'shame' among analysts, who despite years of analysis, continued to 'act out' and behave neurotically (Etchegoyen, 1991; Hopkins, 2008; Aguayo, 2011).

Little (1951, p. 33) highlighted the unconscious nature of countertransference which 'cannot be observed directly … but only in its effects'. This was an obvious but important point: trying 'to observe and interpret something unconscious in oneself is rather like trying to see the back of one's own head – it is a lot easier to see the back of someone else's' (*ibid*.). The 'effects' here might take various forms: the analyst drifting off into seemingly irrelevant fantasy, annoyance, or parentally protective postures towards the patient, or acting out (e.g. stopping sessions early or 'forgetting' to inform a patient about a holiday arrangement). Little was an early proponent of the idea of an intersubjective aspect of countertransference; also its specificity:

> ... it will always include something which is specific to both the individual patient and the individual analyst. That is, every counter-transference is different from every other.
>
> *Little (1951, p. 33)*

This foreshadows Ogden's (1994) description of the 'analytic third' – a uniquely created element between patient and analyst, never to be repeated, but which recreates elements from the past in the present and which 'belong' to neither, and both, analyst and patient.

Money-Kyrle (1956) describes 'normal' countertransference which takes the form of the analytic dyad as a repetition of the parent–child dyad. The analyst operates in an 'oscillation between introjections and projection' (*ibid*., p. 361), where the analyst may become 'introjectively identified' with the patient and will then 're-project him and interpret' (*ibid*.). This takes the theorisation of projective identification another step in the direction of mutuality: the patient's 'projective identification' contributes to 'the analyst's disturbed emotions', which will in turn have an effect on the patient (*ibid*., p. 365).

Countertransference and projective identification: Bion's contribution

At this point a detour is necessary into Klein's (1946) notion of projective identification. This can be defined as:

> a defence mechanism used by the early ego in states of anxiety when, in an omnipotent phantasy, it splits off and projects parts of itself into the object with consequent identifications for ego and object that structure their ensuing relations.
>
> *Spillius & O'Shaughnessy (2012, p. xx)*

Heimann's formulations implied that countertransference could include the projective identifications of the patient. Unpublished archival material shows that Klein herself had suggested that countertransference could be a product of projective processes transferred from patient to analyst (Hinshelwood, 2008).

Spillius (1996a) suggests that Klein was worried that this new understanding of countertransference as coming from the patient would lead to analysts blaming their own deficiencies on their patients. For her, projective identification is interactive. It can be used 'to control the object, to acquire its attributes, to evacuate a bad quality, to protect a good quality, to avoid separation' (1996b, p. 83). Spillius (*ibid.*, p. 10), points out that 'unlike Klein ... [Bion] was explicitly prepared to use his own feelings as a source of information about what the patient was doing'.

With Bion (1959) the interactive aspect of projective identification is explicitly developed. Bion's prototype is the mother's response to the projective identifications of the baby. Emotional engagement is essential, the analyst/mother must be able to take on the feeling, to introject and in a sense 'become' the suffering baby. But the introjection must not be overwhelming. It is processed, and 'handed back' in more manageable form:

> the infant projectively disavows affects and internal states that are intolerable and thus facilitates their containment by the mother. These feelings are 'detoxified' and metabolised by the mother and reinternalized by the infant, who is able to experience them more fully through means of identification with the mother. *Bion was explicit in stressing that an interpersonal interaction occurs above and beyond the projector's unconscious fantasy.*
>
> *Gabbard (1995, p. 476; emphasis added)*

Bion's model is of a to-and-fro process in which unconscious feelings and phantasies flow between mother and baby. This picture can be applied to psychotherapists' countertransference as it is stimulated or aroused by the patient's projections. But if projective identification is interpersonal and interactive, projections can flow either way – not just, as is normally the case, from child to parent, but also vice versa. Segal (1977) suggests that children who have, in this way, been objects of excessive parental projections, as patients may induce in analysts feelings of helplessness in relation to these projections – i.e. here the patient is 'identified' with the projecting parent, the analyst with the child as receptacle of parental projections without resources to 'metabolise' them. The infant's/patient's anxiety needs to be 'modified by having been contained', leading eventually to an object 'capable of containing and dealing with anxiety' being introjected (Segal, 1975, p. 134).

Rosenfeld (1952, p. 117) notes that especially in the analysis of psychotic patients who have 'great verbal difficulties' the 'unconscious intuitive understanding' of the analyst becomes all the more important. Through this 'evocative projective identification' the patient's projections evoke feelings in the analyst which are part of his countertransference and which help in his understanding of the patient's unformulated and often tormented inner world.

As a caveat, Spillius notes that it is possible for the analyst to be 'over preoccupied with monitoring their own feelings ... to the detriment of their direct contact with their patient's material' (1996b, p. 10). This may represent a necessary caution – the analyst's focus must always be on the patient, and only on those aspects of her own feelings that are stimulated or evoked by the patient's projections. Brenman Pick's answer to this dilemma is that the analyst must be able to experience disturbance and respond 'with interpretation that does not convey disturbing anxiety' (Brenman Pick, 1985, p. 157).

Joseph Sandler

Building on Bion's (1959) notion that in the process of projection the projector induces feelings in the projectee that are in line with the projector's phantasy, Sandler (1976) developed his theory of 'role responsiveness'. The projector 'casts' the projectee in a role' (e.g. 'loving mother', 'punitive father' etc.); the projectee then 'responds' by initially unconsciously fulfilling the projector's phantasies by enacting that role. In analysis, awareness of that process (the analyst 'feels' himself being pulled to play a particular role) can then be put to therapeutic advantage. The recipient will feel pressure to act on the projected feelings.

In Sandler's conception, 'transference' is an inherently relational phenomenon, and therefore transference and countertransference are interactive. This may include the role in which the patient casts him or herself 'and a complementary role in which he casts the analyst' (*ibid.*, p. 44). This is incorporated into analytic technique as 'free floating responsiveness' (p. 45) – the analyst needs to be open to these shaping processes if he/she is to enter into the interactive force field created by the patient's unconscious processes.

Attempting perhaps to distance himself from the Kleinian school, Sandler (1976) rejects the notion of projective identification as providing a full explanation for role responsiveness, insisting instead on it as a mutual, normal and healthy creation. Role responsiveness relates to the fundamental processes of empathy, mirroring and 'primary identification' by which people come to know one another, and especially how mothers respond to their babies' feelings and actions.

To conclude this part of the discussion, it is hard to discern much difference between Bion's 'object relations' model of interactive projective identification and Sandler's role responsiveness (see Midgley, 2003). Money-Kyrle (1956), Sandler (1976) and Grinberg (1979) all highlight the importance of the analyst observing his or her own feelings as a guide to those of the patient, particularly feelings of therapeutic impotence or protectiveness. In these formulations, projective processes are accessed via the analyst's emotional response to the patient, i.e. through internal monitoring of his or her inner feeling states. Countertransference is 'unconscious' but can be made conscious through inner 'free floating attention' and self-observation on the part of the analyst. Once these feelings are recognised it is possible to monitor the extent to which the behaviour might reflect what the patient unconsciously seeks to induce in the object, thereby opening up new potential lines of understanding.

The following chapter expands on the contribution of Bion and his followers in formulating analytic subjectivity.

Note

1 Compare this with 'counterpoint' in music, which involves the relationship between voices that are interdependent harmonically and thematically but independent in rhythm and tone.

3

BION AND BEYOND

Reverie was Bion's dream-child. So let's now return to his ideas in an attempt to relate the varying uses of countertransference, projective identification and role responsiveness to his concept, and prefigure how they might be relevant to research.

Bion immerses the reader in a psychoanalytic understanding of reverie with a two-page exposition in his book *Learning from Experience*, where the word appears 14 times (*ibid.*, pp. 36–37). Introducing his book, he states that 'it may seem that I am mis-using words with an established meaning … I have deliberately used them … and I wish the ambiguity to remain' (p. iv). Consistent with a stance of 'learning from experience', the *reverie* word is intriguingly sprung upon the reader in quite shocking ways, with no explanation or definition:

> Leaving aside the physical channels of communication my impression is that her [mother's] love is expressed by reverie.
>
> ibid. *(pp. 35–36)*

This description may lead the reader to believe that Bion was arguing that reverie is the expression of the loving mother 'processing' her infant's mental communications. Just as physical components like milk require digestion, so do mental ones, and mother's reverie provides this metaphorical 'digestion'. Breast and milk are useless to the infant without an alimentary canal to convert them into nourishment. Similarly, the muddling, invading psycho-somatic feelings of the baby will be evacuated without processing (and therefore inaccessible for integrating into emotional experience) if the mother in that moment is incapable of 'sitting with them', digesting them and 'feeding them back', through soothing caresses or words. Bion encapsulates these interactive processes as 'reverie', which he later incorporated into his quasi-mathematical term 'alpha function' (Bion, 1962a, 1970).

Elements of the 'daydreaming' aspect of reverie are also present in Bion's reformulation of the word. He describes reverie as spontaneous and effortless. Reverie, like dreams, and love, cannot be forced. But instead of communicating introspective and self-centred dreaming, reverie now becomes the means by which mother expresses her love for her baby.

For Bion (1962b), reverie is what helps adults understand infants' minds. Etchegoyen (1991, p. 588) suggests that Bion reformulated projective identification as communicative. The mother's reverie is the psychic receiver of the baby's projection; reverie and projection are in constant relational flux. As well as putting forward this communicative aspect of projective identification, it is also no longer linked with psychopathology and is normalised with Bion's model. If the infant's

> intolerance of frustration reaches beyond a certain degree, omnipotent mechanisms come into operation, notably projective identification. This might still be regarded as *realistic*, in that it suggests awareness of the value of a capacity for thought as a means of softening frustration when the reality principle is dominant.
>
> *Bion (1962b, p. 37, emphasis added)*

In other words, the infant 'knows' the mother is there for him or her, to help soothe and process overwhelming feelings.

In Bion's model it is unclear whether reverie is a purely unconscious, spontaneous phenomenon, or whether it also contains conscious willed elements – or indeed whether it could be conscious but still 'unwilled'. Here Bion is ambiguous:

> If the feeding mother cannot allow reverie or if the reverie is allowed but is not associated with love for the child or its father this fact will be communicated to the infant even though incomprehensible to the infant.
>
> ibid. *(p. 37)*

This seems to imply both that reverie is a spontaneous phenomenon, but also that there is a degree of choice as to whether it is 'allowed' or permitted to rise to the surface, and whether it is accompanied by love. Given that psychoanalysis is a 'treatment' for various forms of psychological disturbance, we see Bion wrestling here with a healthy/pathological dichotomy, depending on whether reverie can or cannot surface in the mother's mind, and whether or not it is 'associated with love' (incapacity for loving being a manifestation of psychopathology).

This confusion about the conscious aspect of reverie is noted by Hess (2000, p. 270) as he contrasts Bion's and Ogden's conceptions of reverie. He describes the latter as 'a much more conscious activity' (*ibid.*) than Bion's. Furthermore, reading Bion it is not clear *what* is or is not being 'allowed': whether it is the reverie itself, or its contents such as resentment or even hatred. Nor is it clear exactly what it is about reverie which provides the containment needed for the projector's feelings to be modulated – the empathic reception/resonance on the part of the mother in itself, or her capacity to think about the feelings that have been transmitted or evoked in her.

Bion does offer a loose clarification of reverie:

> that state of mind which is open to the reception of any "objects" from the loved object and is therefore capable of reception of the infant's projective identifications whether they are felt by the infant to be good or bad.
>
> *Bion (1962b, p. 36)*

This suggests a mother who can cope with the 'bad' projections of her baby, i.e. to not be overwhelmed by or rejecting of them, but remains reflective:

> a mother in a state of reverie accepts her infant's projective identifications by sustaining their impact without being transformed by them.
>
> *Grotstein (1984, p. 104)*

For Bion, reverie contains within it its original meaning of dreaming, in the sense of being unwilled, unconscious and 'creative', but, importantly, 'dreaming' now becomes an ongoing daytime as well as a night-time process. Pistiner de Cortinas (2011, p. 136) highlights the dreaming/digesting metaphor: just as night-time 'dream-work' consists of 'digesting' the 'day's residue', so the mother's reverie helps digest the infant's fragmented experiences. Bion's reverie moves from a theory of mother–infant relationship to one of dreaming itself, in which the dream itself acts like a mother 'containing' and allowing work on hitherto unprocessed daytime experiences, as well as the childhood traumata to which they are linked and which they evoke.

The paradox of reverie: 'inward-facing' communication

For Bion reverie denotes the flow of feelings between mother and baby, and, by analogy, analyst and analysand. But caution is called for. We dream alone, albeit immersing ourselves in our 'inner object relations'. If reverie is a waking dream, how can it be usefully thought of as relational? Indeed, the (possibly tautologous) phrase 'autistic reverie' (e.g. Chessick, 1982, p. 160) has been used. Ron Britton describes this difficulty, probably half-jokingly, during a public discussion:

> I don't like this term "reverie". I have a sensitivity to language and the implications of words. I think it may be used to describe a receptive state, but it never sounds to me like a receptive state and I wouldn't like to be received by somebody in the reverie. I think I would rather have their attention.
>
> *Britton et al. (2006, p. 306)*

Britton's objection could be seen in terms of a two-phase model. The first step towards reverie is a focused attention – Winnicott's (1965b) 'primary maternal preoccupation' – followed by the loosened, dreamy state of mind in which infant affect can be contained and thought about. The concept seems to encompass both an 'autistic' breakdown in relating and 'a trance state of optimal receptivity to impulses from within and from the external world with a minimum of defensiveness' (Grotstein (1995, p. 398). This suggests an inherent, but possibly creative, paradox in the idea of reverie: both an inward self-absorption and a below-consciousness communication between mother and child, or analyst and patient. Without 'dreaming' in the Bionian, communicative sense of reverie, communication is 'deadened' (Ogden, 1997c, p. 724), but if all we do is to dream, we lose touch with reality, including the reality of the other.

For Etchegoyen, reverie is 'that state where the spirit allows itself to be led by its memories and imaginings' (Etchegoyen, 1991, p. 588). Etchegoyen wonders why Bion used the word 'reverie' rather than 'maternal care' and suggests this was because he aspired

> to reach another level – perhaps a more abstract, more subjective, more psychological one ... what Bion wishes to emphasize is ... the inter-subjective emotional contact, which gives the mother / child relationship significance.
>
> *Etchegoyen (1991, p. 589)*

The poetic, unexpected, and inexplicable is implicit in Bion's choice and timing of words. The term reverie is uncompromisingly psychoanalytic; 'maternal care' has detached, hygienist, rational, positivist overtones. For Bion, reverie was more than mere daydreaming. With his arts background which preceded his medical training he may well have been influenced by Coleridge's description of creativity, where poetry is composed 'without any sensation of consciousness of effort' (Coleridge, cited in Sharples, 1999, p. 50).

Bion's idea of communicative reverie can be applied to the interplay between producers and receivers of aesthetic objects. The artist's reverie is necessary in generating the artwork, which in turn induces a parallel 'dream-state' in the receiver, or an 'imaginative recreation' (Glover, 2009, p. xiv). The power of art is the 'awakening of emotional communication' (Bajc, 2011). The dream state of the artist 'gets inside' or is embodied in the artwork, and is reawakened for each person who experiences it (Harris Williams, 2010). It is clearly hard to resist turning extensively to the artistic phrases and constructions of other writers; for example, as the novelist Saul Bellow describes, 'True poise, that of contemplation or imagination, sits right on the border of sleep and dreaming' (1975, p. 306).

Artworks which replicate reality may be technically admirable, but may not awaken or come from the dream-life (Weir, 1996). The impressionist movement arose among artists attempting to recreate the ever-changing play of light on the rivers Seine and Oise (Adams, 1990). Instead of aiming to accurately recreate reality, the painters sought to capture flux – both externally (as the sun moves in the sky, and the river flows) and internally. Their vision of the world, a species of reverie, was tied up with their emotions in the moment of creation.

We shall see later how this emphasis on the creative aspects of reverie is relevant to researchers' efforts to approach participants with spontaneity and creativity, and how artistic expression can be used in RRM training groups to induce reverie-related states of mind.

Post-Bionian elaborations

Bion's abstract minimalism meant that he did not elaborate a coherent theory of reverie so much as tantalising and disconnected ideas. Others have picked up the pieces and the process of theory-building is ongoing (e.g. Ogden, 1997b; Bollas, 1998; Ferro, 2002; Birksted-Breen, 2012). These authors, in different ways, place reverie at the centre of analytic work, i.e. understanding unconscious interpersonal communication.

Ferro and Ogden both develop the idea of 'waking dreaming'. Stars continue to shine in the sky, despite being obscured by the light of day (Ogden, 2001). For Ogden, and Ferro, dreaming is 'a continuous process that takes place in waking life as well as in sleep' (Ferro, 2002, p. 597). If reverie is (day-) dreaming then we are all the time dreaming, whether or not asleep, and there exists the constant potential for entering a reverie state of mind, with degrees and varieties of defensive blockades needing to be overcome in order to access these states of mind. Ogden (2003) and Ferro (2011) suggest that reverie should be used to refer not to daydreams as such, but to those moments when a person is in contact with his or her normally obscured waking dream thought processes. In this sense reverie is a description of the unconscious in action – silently shaping our thoughts and actions, but mostly out of conscious awareness. In addition, the term reverie can refer either to the *state* of receptivity to waking dream thought, and/or the *content* of this receptivity. In other words, reverie can refer to both a state of mind and the imagistic contents of the mind at any given moment.

According to Grotstein (1979, p. 144) 'the dream is therapy in a dramatic form', and the psychic importance of dreaming is encapsulated in his conception of the 'dreaming couple'. While Freud thought that dreams had to be 'unpacked' (with dream thoughts jammed together like 'pack-ice', Freud, 1900, p. 312) to be made comprehensible, for Bion the material 'has to be subjected to *dreamwork* to render it suitable for storing away and for thought' (Ferro, 2002, p. 598, emphasis added). In other words, the dream has to be 're-dreamed' by the listener, just as the mother 'dreams' her baby's dream-life. For Bion, this 'dreamwork' is the maternal function.

Translating the mother–infant pair into adult life, the 'dreaming couple' comprises a 'Dreamer Who Dreams the Dream' and a 'Dreamer Who Understands the Dream', the former corresponding to the projections of the infant, and the latter to the mother's capacity for reverie (Grotstein, 1979, p. 115). The latter could be the healthy, mature or 'well-analysed' dreamer him or herself, or the analyst.

> Dreaming is the absorption and transformation of internal and external sensual data which, after they have been 'dreamed', are then ready for mental digestion.
>
> ibid., *pp. 115–116*

This is a three-way process, since, in good-enough circumstances, the infant then re-introjects the mother's capacity for reverie and grows up to be someone who is both able to dream and to mentally digest dream content. Relevant to this model are findings from infant observation research which emphasise the two-way elements of the development of the infant's personality, in which the infant influences the style of maternal provision, and vice versa, rather than a unidirectional influence (mother to infant) as was previously visualised (Trevarthen & Aitken, 2001; Beebe et al., 2005).

Narrative derivatives

If there is a continuity of 'dreaming' in this Bionian sense between night-time and waking life, then, in Ferro's model, our words and actions can be seen as 'narrative derivatives' (Ferro, 2002; Civitarese, 2008; Civitarese & Ferro, 2013) of dream processes:

> The seriation of α elements making up the process of continuous formation of waking dream thought has an infinite number of possible narrative derivatives.
>
> *Ferro (2002, p. 600)*

Patient responses to the analyst or the analytic situation are 'narrative derivatives of waking dream thought' (*ibid.*, p. 589). For Ferro, working with narrative derivatives is the basis of psychoanalytic interpretation. A patient's description of something 'outside' the analysis ('my friend's car broke down') or concrete ('I want to know what days your holidays are') may be seen as communications concerning dream thoughts. In response to the above the analyst might think or 'interpret': 'our analysis isn't getting anywhere; it's broken down'; or 'I am anticipating the feeling of being left, alone, with no one to hold me, like an abandoned baby'.

For Ferro (2002) everyday conversation – which could also include research interviews – contains 'narrative derivatives' of these unconscious thoughts. I shall show how in the RRM the interviewer's reverie is used to capture the themes that give rise to the participant's narrative derivatives.

Reverie versus countertransference

Implicit in Bion's conception of reverie is the importance of not-knowing, i.e. Keatsian 'negative capability':

> The mother gradually dispels the baby's distress, seeking to engage with it *rather than to explain* it. She is able to tolerate *not knowing its source* … she gently talks, rocks, strokes, feeds, reflects, until her baby, basking in the calm of trustful intimacy, begins to recover.
>
> *Waddell (2000, p. 30, emphasis added)*

This contrasts with the pre-Heimann countertransference, i.e. outside of conscious control, and arising out of the analyst's blind spots, as in Freud's original public concept of countertransference. In Ferro and Ogden's extensions of the Bion model, reverie reflects the continuous workings of the unconscious, whether one is awake or asleep. Classical countertransference is a subset of reverie, referring to the analyst's complexes and traumata insofar as they are aroused by contact with the patient. Heimann's countertransference is yet another subset, the projections of the patient as they are picked up and contained by the analyst's unconscious.

We can now define 'relational reverie': a further subset within the wider context of reverie, containing elements of both classical and projectively driven Heimannian countertransference, but distinct from both. *Relational reverie refers to an interactive, interpsychic mutual resonance between analyst and patient.*

Relational reverie thus defined is achieved through consciously ('purposively') engaging with the patient and his or her 'material' – i.e. dream thoughts – but in an 'evenly-suspended' (Freud, 1912, p. 111) way. Negative capability denotes the receptiveness implicit in relational reverie: the sense of having 'all the time in the world' (Ogden 2005a, p. 1272), and that there is 'no need to account for the "value" of each session' (Ogden, 1995, p. 570).

In Bion's model, the capacity for reverie, and negative capability itself, imply a capacity which presents in parents and analysts to a greater or lesser extent, and which in theory is enhanced by psychoanalytic training. For Winnicott (1971) analysis was learning to play; for Bion, and in turn Ogden and Ferro, it may be about enhancing the capacity for mutual dreaming. Winnicott (1971, p. 38) saw 'psychotherapy taking place in the overlap of two areas of playing', while for Ogden (1997b, p. 568) it is based on 'overlapping states of reverie'. The ability to 'dream' in this Bionian sense chimes with the playfulness of the analytic pair. An analytic session is an exercise in mutual and playful reverie.

For Winnicott, 'creative receptivity', a state akin to reverie, is the essential precursor ('the only basis') for 'self-discovery and a sense of existing' (Winnicott, 1971, p. 82). Winnicott's being/doing dichotomy parallels the receptive–creative polarity at the centre of the theory of reverie. The receptive element is the necessary first step, the 'being' element; then, later, comes the 'doing', the capacity to put things into words, or (especially in child analysis) actively to play. But without this initial 'being', creative 'doing' could not happen.

Privacy and reverie

Winnicott (1971 p. 98) famously said of the game of hide-and-seek, 'it is a joy to be hidden and a disaster not to be found'.

> Although healthy persons communicate and enjoy communicating, the other fact is equally true, that each individual is an isolate, permanently non-communicating, permanently unknown, in fact, unfound ... At the centre of each

> person is an incommunicado element, and this is sacred and most worthy of preservation.
>
> *Winnicott (1963, p. 187)*

Reverie is an 'attempt to reach an area that has no words' (Weir, 1996, p. 327). Ogden (1996) suggests that respecting privacy, for both analyst and patient, is essential for reverie. Over-enthusiastic incitement of patients to freely associate goes against this: 'it is as important for a patient to know that he is free to be silent as it is for him to know that he is free to speak (*ibid.*, p. 889).

Favouring speaking over silence, or disclosure over privacy, may violate the principles of reverie. Silence here refers both to literal absence of noise, but also the space for inner reflection. We cannot talk from our hearts if we cannot be silent. Silence may be emotionally communicative (Olinick, 1982, Leira, 1995). In those moments when we feel compelled to speak, speech interrupts dreaming. In music, silence – rests, pauses, beginnings, endings – and the intervening sounds each need to be 'heard' in relation to one another. The RRM aims to balance respect for privacy and silence against the revelatory aspect of the researcher's reverie.

Reverie as communication: Ogden and the analytic 'third'

We shall look in detail at Ogden's contribution to the concept of reverie and its relevance to the RRM in Chapter 5. But to anticipate, here is a brief clinical excerpt:

> As she led the way from the waiting room into the consulting room, I could feel in my body the patient's drinking in of every detail of the hallway. I noticed several small flecks of paper from my writing pad on the carpet. I *knew* that the patient was taking them in and hoarding them "inside" of her to silently dissect mentally during and after the session.
>
> *Ogden (1997b, p. 572, emphasis in original)*

Reverie 'takes the most mundane, personal, and private of shapes, often involving the minutiae of everyday life' (Ogden, 1997b, p. 567). Receptiveness, attending to changes in body states and sensory perceptions, facilitates speaking from the 'groundedness' of emotional experience (*ibid.*, p. 568). For Ogden there is a contextual, here-and-now, unique mutually derived 'third' in all analytic relationships which is distinct from the inner world or unconscious of patient ('first'), or analyst ('second'). Ogden's analytic third 'stands in dialectical tension with the analyst and analysand as separate individuals with their own subjectivities' (1996, p. 884).

In relational reverie, the psychoanalyst 'loses' himself or herself through a concentrated focus on the patient. The analytic situation is 'asymmetrical' in 'privileging … the exploration of the unconscious life of the analysand' (i.e. not that of the analyst) (*ibid.*). Conceptualised in terms of the intersubjectively created third, the analyst does not lose him or herself 'in' the patient's psyche, but, rather, both together lose themselves in the jointly created yet uniquely experienced third space.

If a dream is not seen as 'belonging' to the patient, or analyst, but as an 'intersubjective analytic event' (Ogden, 1996, p. 892), the analytic third provides a new way of viewing projective identification:

> now projection, instead [of] being understood as directed into the object, can be seen as projected half way, into an intermediate potential space felt by the analysand as indistinguishable from the analyst.
>
> *Grotstein (2000, p. 630)*

Conclusion

For the purposes of the RRM model to be developed later, imagine a Venn diagram. Reverie is the biggest or 'outer' circle. Within it lies countertransference, both the analyst's 'own' projections (classical 'Freudian' countertransference) and projectively identified patient-derived elements (Heimannian countertransference). To these I would add a third ('Ogdonian') overlapping zone between the two, where relational responses arise in the mind of the analyst, evoked and resonating with the patient.

This chapter has described the analyst's use of his/her own subjectivity, affect and relationally induced reverie as a means, possibly the prime means, of deepening psychoanalytic understanding. Ever since Freud's early letters on the subject of countertransference, this has been a contentious issue. Given Freud's championing of the dream as the 'royal road' to the unconscious, and that dreaming and reverie are etymologically and conceptually equivalent, the role of reverie in psychoanalysis has been lying latent for some time. The early literature on countertransference lacked the conceptual ingredient brought by Bion – communicative projective identification, and by implication, communicat*ed* countertransference.

The previous chapters have explored how the analyst's subjectivity has been understood psychoanalytically. Whether seen in terms of projective identification, or from a more intersubjective perspective, there is increasing agreement that the analyst's subjective responses can be used at a clinical level as a method of 'research' (Heimann, 1950, p. 81) into the other's unconscious, and/or the unconscious intersubjective dynamic. The next chapter both shows and critiques how systematic psychoanalytically oriented research attempts to draw on these ideas in order to develop reflexive research strategies.

4

REVERIE, REFLEXIVITY AND RESEARCH INTERVIEWS

We are now beginning to move in a research direction. In this chapter I shall introduce the role of RRM in qualitative research, starting with an outline of the theoretical background to qualitative research interviewing. Next, the growing interest in researcher reflexivity is examined. I touch on ways in which psychoanalytic theory has been drawn on by qualitative researchers, especially in the notion of 'subjectivity' as developed in the previous chapters. Some of the problematics of qualitative approaches to research interviews are delineated, before describing how the RRM may respond to them.

The What and How of Qualitative Research

The advent of 'qualitative' research paradigms in the social and psychological sciences is relatively recent (Denzin & Lincoln, 2011). In some ways a 'qualitative/quantitative' research distinction is artificial and misleading. For example, quantitative approaches are usually seen to be strong on generalisability, while qualitative approaches are renowned for close-up, experiential understandings, especially in investigating single cases. However, several authors have argued that case studies, no less than quantitative research, can yield generalisable knowledge (e.g. Flyvbjerg, 2006; Hinshelwood, 2010). For example, Hinshelwood (2010, p. 371) suggests that a single case – the so-called 'black swan paradigm' – can falsify a hypothesis if there is: '(a) a clear binary question, and (b) one counter-example to demolish it'. It only took one Columbus to demolish the hypothesis that the world was flat (*ibid.*), and only one black swan to prove that not all swans are white.

Silverman (2013) outlines the features usually thought of as 'qualitative', which include:

- open questions that do not lend themselves to numerical answers (Liamputtong, 2009; Flick, 2014);
- a small numbers of participants (Sandelowski, 1995; Crouch & McKenzie, 2006);
- exploring human behaviour and motivations (Bogdan & Biklen, 1982);
- case-study stimulus – i.e. research arising out of clinical practice leading to 'practice-based evidence' (Eisenhardt, 1989; Green & Latchford, 2012);
- studying phenomena in the contexts in which they arise, in naturalistic rather than laboratory-like conditions;
- 'backwards' methodology – i.e. research questions which are generated from the research process itself, or in the midst of data analysis, rather than pre-determining the analysis;
- links to an ethical or philosophical position which determines how data will be collected and interpreted.

Examples of the latter include ethnography (Clifford & Marcus, 1986; Willis & Trondman, 2000), grounded theory (Glaser, 1978); phenomenology (Giorgi, 1985; Merleau-Ponty, 1962), and discourse analysis (Avdi, 2008). This methodological diversity is an inevitable outcome of something which is inherently hard to define; however, it can also lead to qualitative research becoming factional, especially if an investigation becomes overly driven by a particular theoretical position (this is a potential critique which could be levelled at the RRM!).

If the essence of qualitative research is *the study of humans under human conditions*, a possible unifying theme is the sense of a research focus emerging in a spontaneous, unplanned but phenomenologically responsive way. Research infrastructure (for example, Dictaphones, consent forms, interview schedules) may no doubt be needed, but can also interfere with this 'naturalistic' objective. Implicit in a philosophically flexible approach to researching, how to conduct qualitative research would not be predetermined, and could be tailored to the specifics of the research question and/or the phenomena under investigation.

Exploring qualitative approaches further, research interviews are by far the most common qualitative research strategy, perhaps even becoming a 'go to' method, with insufficient critical evaluation about its suitability (Potter & Hepburn, 2005). Interviews have been estimated to have been used for data collection in 90 per cent of social science investigations (Briggs, 1986). Silverman (2013) suggests a similar figure in his examination of one edition of a qualitative journal, where 16 out of 18 studies used interviews.

Given this prevalence, the methodology of research interviewing has been extensively discussed among scholars (e.g. Mishler, 1991; Wengraf, 2001; Gubrium & Holstein, 2001; Gillham, 2005; Kvale & Brinkmann, 2008; Edwards & Holland, 2013). The research interview usually involves a number of components. A researcher meets with a participant. The researcher aims to get a sense of the participant's thoughts and feelings about a research topic (e.g. 'migration' or 'bereavement'). Sampling is often 'purposeful': the participants will have been selected because they have some degree of personal experience of the topic. There is explicit recognition of the value of a personalised and unique perspective offered by an 'expert by experience'. The general view about how researchers 'get a sense' of the participant's experience is through asking open-ended, but often 'semi-structured' (i.e. predetermined, but flexible as to order, phraseology, etc.), questions, as well as statements or other cues such as head-nodding encouraging the participant to respond.

Research interviewing has two interlinked components – conducting the interview itself, and interpreting the 'results' of the interview, in a process named 'data analysis' (Scheurich, 1997).

Why the interview has become the dominant method of researching is to an extent self-evident, although its selection as a method can sometimes lack sufficient research pre-planning (Potter & Hepburn, 2005). While naturalistic, observational studies flow freely, an interview methodology is more controlled, and so can be more focused on a 'research question' and be 'participant-centred' (Riach, 2009, p. 356). Interviews provide greater depth and subtlety than standard self-report measures and questionnaires, which fail to capture freedom of individual expression and nuance, where participants can voice their stories in an unstructured way. An interview is a 'conversation with a purpose' (Schaeffer, 1991, p. 34), so has the further advantage of being interactive. The researcher can ask for in-the-moment clarification, question further, probe and so on. Later, if, as is usual, the interview has been recorded, there is an opportunity for 'immersion' in the data: listening, re-listening, transcribing and reflecting on what has transpired (Ritchie & Spencer, 2002, p. 179; Thorne, 2000).

'Subjectivity' in qualitative research

Given that psychoanalysis can also be seen as a 'conversation' between analyst and analysand (Barkham et al. 2017), there is an overlap between qualitative research theory and psychoanalytic ideas, especially those that concentrate on intersubjectivity. Interviews are increasingly conceptualised as interactional (Silverman, 2013) and collaboratively produced (Gubrium & Holstein, 2004). Interview guidelines and training skills focus on rapport-building (Rapley, 2004), 'trying to interact with that specific person' (*ibid.*, p. 25), calling to mind the 'therapeutic alliance' in psychotherapy.

There is however a tension between the need to be 'participant-led', which produces gains in authenticity, but may remain superficial, and those in which the researcher asks probing questions, but may thereby impose a predetermined theoretical agenda, rather than allowing for the spontaneous emergence of novelty and surprise. Interviews which aim to be participant-centred, but without researcher-led probes, may lack richness and complexity. It would also be a misconception to believe that deeper meaning emerges *exclusively* through asking more and more probing questions.

The RRM is an attempt to move beyond this dilemma of true-to-participant authenticity versus interviewer-guided depth. The RRM views the interview as an interactional dialogue in which the data arise as much in the responsive mind of the interviewer as it does in the words of the participant. Researcher subjectivity, rather than being potentially contaminating, now becomes a source of research information. But – a crucial question – can this data be reliably and systematically gathered and analysed?

The idea of internal reflection as a data source is developed in the literature on researcher 'reflexivity' (Finlay & Gough, 2003). In this 'turn', researchers are encouraged to think about their own role vis-à-vis participants (Ellis & Bochner, 2000; Mauthner & Doucet, 2003; Finlay, 2002a, 2002b; Finlay & Gough, 2003; Etherington, 2004). Just as there was a *volte face* in how countertransference was viewed in psychoanalysis, so what was previously perceived as the 'problem' of subjectivity in research now becomes an opportunity.

In a research context, reflexivity is defined as 'thoughtful, self-aware analysis of the intersubjective dynamics between researcher and researched' (Finlay & Gough, (2003, p. ix). Reflexivity has come to be seen as important in qualitative research because the researcher is the primary instrument for collecting and interpreting data. This introduction of 'thoughtfulness', 'self-awareness' and 'intersubjectivity' into the qualitative research arena may open a window for reverie-informed researching. The RRM aims to strike a balance between being 'inward turned' (accessing reverie through observing one's subjective responses), while also 'being there' in the moment and interactively engaged with the participant.

As a backdrop to the RRM, let us examine in more detail some qualitative research ventures that have been influenced by psychoanalytic ideas.

Psychoanalytically informed research strategies

Attempting to overcome concern about the emotional 'distance' (Michael Rustin, 2003, p. 140) between researchers and participants which arises as an outcome of some traditional research approaches, qualitative researchers have been drawn to psychoanalysis. Psychoanalysis involves 'close-up', personalised methods of understanding subjects. Freud (1912, p. 114) claimed that in psychoanalysis 'research and treatment coincide'. This has been taken as inspiration not just for psychoanalysts – often to their detriment to the extent that they have neglected systematic research – but as a way in which qualitative researchers might capture more nuanced interactive phenomenology (e.g. Pile, 1991; Kvale, 1999; Shamai, 2003; Gough, 2004; Midgley, 2006a, 2006b; Rizq, 2008; Branney, 2008).

In line with the reflexive turn, and the valuation of subjectivity, researchers have explored parallels between the 'analytic dyad' (Bourdeau, 2000) and the 'research dyad'. In this comparison, the researcher is compared with the psychoanalyst, and the participant is in a similar position to the patient (Kvale, 1999; Cartwright, 2004; Melles, 2005; Drisko, 2004; Lewis, 2008). Contributions to this field include Devereux's (1967) and Hunt's (1989) arguments that unconscious processes in the researcher shape their research strategies. Devereux's was probably the first exposition of 'researcher countertransference', depicting an inevitably non-neutral researcher, tied up with a host of competing and unconscious motivations and defences. Here were prototype visions of psychoanalytically informed researcher reflexivity.

In addition to reflexivity, psychoanalytic understandings of emotional defences have also entered the qualitative research field. Focusing primarily on participant rather than researcher defensiveness, Hollway & Jefferson pioneered the 'free association narrative interview' (Hollway & Jefferson, 2000; see also Gadd, 2004; Osofsky & Osofsky, 2009). This is an unstructured interview technique attempting to elicit unconscious material from 'defended subjects'. Their work championed a less restricted interviewing methodology and pointed to anxiety-driven preconceptions which hinder freer researching.

Bringing unconscious processes into consideration means that themes not on pre-planned interview schedules become areas potentially ripe for exploration. Endorsing interviewer–interviewee exploration not confined to preconceptions of the research topic, via encouraging participants' free associations, brought psychoanalytic understandings of defensive processes into the research context, and at the same time highlighted the importance of a spontaneous, 'open to surprise' attitude to research. Less restricted interviewing seems to 'feel right' and has been reported to produce more interesting interviews (Hollway & Jefferson, 2013, pp. 1–4).

This approach entails a realigning of researchers' priorities and ethics. In the first edition (Hollway & Jefferson, 2000), the focus was primarily on the participant's, rather than the researcher's unconscious experiences. This was evident in their attitude towards in-interview 'interpretation'. They advise researchers to be 'careful not to interpret at the time that information is being provided by the interviewee' (Hollway & Jefferson, 2000, p. 77). It was advised that interpretation in research should come in at the stage of 'data analysis as opposed to data production' (*ibid.*). The participant may be encouraged to freely associate but in relation to a researcher who keeps their subjectivity relatively in check. Hollway & Jefferson (2013) later modified their views on in-the-moment 'interpretation' during research interviews. Whether this should be employed 'depends on the many facets of the research situation and the many versions of interpretation' (*ibid.*, p. 157). We shall see later how the RRM approaches this delicate issue of what, when and whether to 'interpret' in relation to research interviews.

Taken together, qualitative research interest in psychoanalysis has crystallised around a new and booming field of academic enquiry: 'psychosocial studies' (Clarke & Hoggett, 2009). This combines close-up, psychoanalytically inspired ideas and techniques with consideration of broader societal influences, especially the power dynamics underlying research topics and methodology.

Researcher reflexivity and psychoanalysis

There have been parallel developments in the domains of psychoanalytic thinking and qualitative research. There is increasing interest in analyst/researcher subjectivity as a means of understanding the other (i.e. patient/participant), as well as the emerging dynamic – the 'third' – which lies between, and emerges out of, these two subjectivities. A number of articles examine researchers' emotional and behavioural responses from a psychoanalytic perspective (Clarke, 2002; Lucey, Melody & Walkerdine, 2003; Marks & Monnich-Marks, 2003; Roper, 2003; Froggett & Wengraf, 2004; Ellis, 2009; Jervis, 2009, 2011; Lorimer, 2010; Morgenroth, 2010; Strømme et al., 2010; Elliott, Ryan & Hollway, 2011; Robben, 2012). These writers have examined the idea that psychic states can be 'transferred' from participant to researcher, in a process analogous to the psychoanalytic concepts of a) 'projection', in which the patient/participant attributes feelings in another as a surrogate for their own emotional states (Freud, 1905) and b) 'projective identification' (Klein, 1946) in which the patient/participant induces – usually unbearable – feelings and sometimes actions in the therapist/researcher.

In research discourse, the phrase 'projective identification' is sometimes used interchangeably with 'countertransference'. However, the 'projective identification' model for understanding how feelings arise in researchers runs the risk of reinforcing an unhelpful power dimension between researcher and researched: 'top down assertion of expert knowledge' (Frosh & Emerson, 2005, p. 322) where 'I, the expert, know that you are unwittingly putting your unbearable feelings into me' (see Frosh & Baraitser, 2008 for further critique).

To summarise the earlier discussion, in the psychoanalytic literature the analyst's subjectivity has been considered in at least three ways: a) *interfering*, classically referring to the muddying elements of the analyst's own neuroses, and as a hindrance to the therapeutic process (e.g. Freud, 1910c); b) *useful*, in which elements of the patient's neurosis are unconsciously transferred onto the analyst, and therefore can help understand the patient's inner world (e.g. Heimann, 1950; Brenman Pick, 1985); c) as *intersubjective and co-created*, containing elements of both a and b (e.g. Ferenczi, 1955 [1928]). This latter sense is the relational 'third' (Ogden, 1994) which cannot be defined exclusively in terms of either analyst or patient, but as product of their interaction. A feeling state or dream that emerges in these conditions 'belongs' neither to the patient nor the analyst (Ogden, 1996), and is understood through consideration of the intersubjective dynamic.

Psychoanalytically minded qualitative researchers have thus far focused mainly on 'useful', 'type b' countertransference (e.g. Jervis, 2009; Lorimer, 2010; Strømme et al,. 2010) based on Heimann's (1950) description of countertransference as an 'instrument of research into the patient's unconscious' (*ibid.*, p. 81). The classic metaphor is that of a resonating tuning fork or telephone receiver (cf. Freud 1912) in which the analyst's receptivity 'picks up' vibrations from the patient's unconscious, thereby providing access to their inner world. A similar process, it is contended, applies to researcher and participant: thus 'countertransference' is transformed into a qualitative research tool.

Clarke (2002) describes how a feeling state or role can be induced in the researcher, suggesting that he was subjected to the 'projective identifications' (p. 174) of his interviewees:

> In the case of Mark's [a participant] interview, we can see processes of both communication and control which I argue Mark uses to create a 'concerned object', to elicit a response in me, in some sense, by controlling my feelings.
>
> *Clarke (2002, p. 185)*

Alternatively, it is contended, when participants' feelings are unbearable, they may be unconsciously projected into the researcher:

> The interviewer's counter-transference reactions indicate those emotions and contents … that interviewees have forgotten, repressed or denied are being re-enacted and projected on the interviewer … who [in] this way is being forced to experience them (counter-transference).
>
> *Marks & Monnich-Marks (2003, no page number, online article)*

Similarly, Strømme et al. (2010, p. 215) argue that through paying attention to

> countertransference reactions and detailing incidents of nonverbal communication [it becomes] possible to draw conclusions about the relational attitude of the participants and their defence processes … Countertransference reactions [may be used] … to gain access to more unconscious processes in the *participant*.
>
> ibid. *(p. 221, emphasis added)*

In each case, the participant's use of projection is fore-fronted while the researcher can remain something of a receptacle. Interviewer 'mistakes' are explained in terms of projective identification, i.e. how the participant induces the researcher to behave in ways that reflects the participant's themes. Nevertheless these authors show awareness of the problem of uni-directionality: 'the psychoanalytically informed research interview represents a certain challenge to the idea of "co-participation" often present in qualitative research' (*ibid.*, p. 221).

In addition to studies which have examined 'useful' countertransference, attempts have also been made to describe 'interfering' countertransference, i.e. the feelings that arise in the researcher that are connected with his or her own past. Such approaches tend to view these two types of countertransference as independent and in need of disentanglement. Lorimer (2010, p. 98) describes 'a case of countertransference that I experienced while doing fieldwork at a Danish psychiatric hospital'. She defines this as a strong sensation in mind or body which 'might indicate the presence of unconscious tension' in the participant (p. 100) (i.e. useful, informative, countertransference understood as projective identification). But later she also recognises the potential for interfering countertransference:

> I had to be aware of whether a mood was brought on by the person I was speaking with or was more obviously connected with an aspect of my own life.
>
> ibid. *(p. 106)*

For Lucey, Melody & Walkerdine (2003, p. 280) researchers' feelings are 'useful indicators of what might be going on for the subjects of the research'. But they also describe how the interviewer's adolescent self was unconsciously activated during an interview with parents about their adolescent child. This shaped the way she responded to her interviewees.

Critique

For psychoanalytically minded qualitative researchers all this is encouraging. Nevertheless, several problems arising from current understandings of researcher subjectivity in the qualitative research literature have been identified.

Problem 1: Approaches which adopt the 'countertransference as projective identification' model reinforce unequal power relations and the myth of the infallible therapist. As briefly mentioned above, several authors (Frosh & Emerson, 2005; Frosh & Baraitser, 2008; Parker, 2010) point out that the view that feelings can be 'put into' the researcher may reinforce an unequal power relationship. Unequal power relations (e.g. Burman, 1992) between researcher and researched have been described in terms of paternalism, class and education. To assume that the feelings of the researcher indicate the state of mind of the participant is

> a direct result of the application of a Kleinian style of psychoanalysis in which the truth of the subject can be known through meditation by (or though the unconscious of) an interlocutor who has more knowledge and understanding than does the subject.
>
> *Frosh & Baraister (2008, p. 363)*

This implies a power imbalance, although it might be argued that researcher and researched are merely adopting differing roles, in which power relations are not relevant. Power differentials may be inevitable (Foucault, 1988), but Winnicott (1969) and others argue that progress is often made through attempting to understand them through psychoanalytic interpretations. Also, the idea that personal analysis will eliminate the therapist's own neurosis, including the desire to exercise power over her patient, takes us back to the early days of psychoanalysis and Freud's search for scientific objectivity (Freud, 1910c). To repeat, Heimann stated in relation to countertransference:

> When the analyst in his own analysis has worked through his infantile conflicts and anxieties ... he will not impute to his patient what belongs to himself.
>
> *Heimann (1950, p. 83)*

Today, it is more usual to acknowledge that even the most well-analysed analysts make mistakes. Likewise, it cannot be correct to assume a fully objective, transparent and self-knowledgeable researcher. More useful for qualitative research may be the intersubjective branches of psychoanalysis, which advocate a stance of analytic 'fallibilism' (Stolorow, 2003, p. 223). When applied to qualitative research this would mean that researchers cannot simply assume that a feeling state has been projected into them, but explore this as one possibility among several.

Problem 2: Pseudo-certainty in understandings of countertransference. Residues of the all-knowing analyst in relation to the distorted views of the patient run the risk of writing with misplaced certainty about research themes derived from countertransference where there is potential for an exploration of multiple and contradictory definitions (see Parker, 2005a, for further critique). Alternatively, the researcher may attempt to resonate in a creative and playful way with the participant's affects, so that new and unexpected meanings are co-created.

Problem 3: Differences between the psychoanalytic and research framework. Despite potentially significant overlaps, research and clinical work are distinct realms. The increasing espousal of countertransference in qualitative research literature may veer towards their conflation (Georgaca, 2005; Parker, 2005b; Frosh & Emerson, 2005; Branney, Gough & Madill, 2009). As Strømme et al. (2010, p. 219, emphasis added) point out, 'since the student therapists [the research participants in their study] had been *asked* to participate in the study, the interviewer had a responsibility to stimulate the interview process'. The authors here make it clear here that the researcher is the initiator, whereas in clinical psychoanalysis it is more usually the patient seeking help who initiates the process. In this sense, the researcher/participant relationship is the antithesis of the therapeutic setting, since it is the *interviewer's* desire which drives the research process, not the other way around (Frosh & Baraitser, 2008).

This has led Frosh & Baraitser (2008, p. 346) to call for a more 'tentative' contribution of psychoanalysis to social research. Similarly, Cartwright (2004) advocates consideration of 'inchoate' transference–countertransference *impressions* in the research setting (p. 221). This might include close observation of changes in the researcher's feeling states, associations and bodily reactions (see e.g. Gemignani, 2011). In before-and-after studies such as the ones to be described later, this could also include the researcher's observations and fantasies about the participant's changes in these domains.

In relation to validation, the qualitative researcher is in some ways in an advantageous position compared to the psychoanalyst. Research data can be cross-compared (e.g. with accounts from participants' relatives, teachers, co-researchers etc.), which would be unethical in the analytic situation. The qualitative researcher is typically free to make use of a Dictaphone for interviews; provide a more flexible frame of interaction (e.g. not having to keep to the 'analytic hour'); and, at the phase of interview transcript analysis, studying it without the immediacy of having to respond to participants in vivo.

'Scenic composition' and social dreaming

Two further examples of creative explorations, which draw on the capacity for reverie, without using this term, both of which have influenced RRM, will now be mentioned. These are the work of Lorenzer and his 'scenic composition' (Bereswill, Morgenroth & Redman, 2010); and Lawrence (2000) on social dreaming.

Lorenzer and scenic composition

Alfred Lorenzer was a German psychoanalyst and Marxist whose aim was to develop a theory and method with which to study the impact of society on the embodied psyche, and, conversely, the influence of deep psychological meanings on social phenomena. His premature death, and the fact that little of his work has been translated into English, mean that it is not as well known as it deserves. Lorenzer developed two RRM-relevant themes: 'scenic understanding' and 'depth hermeneutics'.

'Scenic' refers to an affective register of meaning, with its origins in the early phases of life, operating below the surface and verbal level, yet continuously present. These scenic phenomena are inscribed in the body and brain in the form of 'engrams'. As development proceeds, scenic phenomena typically become symbolised through language – comparable to Ferro's narrative derivatives. But, either through the traumatic nature of experience, or because of social forces antipathetic to symbolisation, this process maybe be aborted or incomplete. Depth hermeneutics then represents the attempt to grasp and recover these unsymbolised scenic understandings/meanings. As Lorenzer puts it:

> The distinguishing feature of psychoanalytical cultural analysis as a 'depth hermeneutic' derives from … the recognition of an autonomous level of meaning below the manifest level present in language … the latent meaning is, in some sense, beyond language but is nevertheless present within it and is consequential in its own right.
>
> *Lorenzer (1986a, p. 29, emphasis in the original, cited in Bereswill, Morgenroth & Redman, 2010 p. 6)*

There are a number of implications of this for the RRM. First, Lorenzer's 'scenic understanding' has clear parallels with Bion and Ogden and Ferro's 'waking dreaming'. The challenge is to find research procedures which tap into this realm. Second, as Hollway (2011) puts it, 'without emotion (or affect) meaning-making is impossible' – again ways to access affect in a systematic research context are needed. Third, if scenic understanding remains unsymbolised, purely verbal research procedures are inadequate for the task – hence, as we shall see, the possibility for alternative research data with researchers' enteroceptive and imagic responses.

Central to Lorenzer's sociological perspective is how social forces impact on scenic understanding. The dominance of instrumental, goal-oriented, 'cognitive' research procedures may mean they inhibit scenic understanding; ways to circumvent this culture need to be found. To this end, Hollway and colleagues (Froggett & Hollway, 2010; Hollway & Froggett, 2012) draw on Lorenzer in attempting to harness researchers' emotional responsiveness. Scenic composition is 'a process by which researchers reflect on their affective and embodied experience of their data'

(Redman, Bereswill, & Morgenroth, 2010, p. 217). Denuded of the feeling content of language, its meaning is impoverished. 'Scenic' understanding aims to provide 'a vivid, visualised rendering of a data extract that preserves its emotional resonance during data analysis and for the reader' (Hollway & Froggett, 2012, no page number, online article).

Here is an example of a scenic composition, describing a research participant:

> Darren is pale, gangly, shaven headed; slouchy shoulders in slouchy, street-cool clothes ... he is childlike – waiting to be led, or entertained, or told what to do. His feet shuffle as if they don't quite belong to him ... Darren rubs his head, stressed.
>
> Ibid.

The aim of the 'scenic composition' is to enable the person to come to life in the mind of the reader, so that it is easier to identify with him, or to 'traverse imaginatively the distance' (*ibid.*) between researcher and participant. This description is full of researcher subjectivity, with imagined feeling states ('Darren rubs his head, stressed'); colloquial and evocative language ('gangly'); emotive, impressionistic – rather than purely descriptive – words ('slouchy, street-cool clothes'). This is a different imaginative creation for the reader in contrast to a standard 'clinical' preamble such as 'Darren is a white 17-year-old from a working-class family in London's East End. He studies computer programming at college.'

Scenic composition aims to capture the emotional atmosphere generated by participant–researcher interaction, typically omitted, or defensively avoided, through conventional demographic descriptions. In later chapters I shall show how the RRM suggests specific ways in which researching this below-surface zone can be achieved and taught.

Lawrence and social dreaming

Social dreaming was 'discovered' by Gordon Lawrence in the 1980s at the Tavistock Institute. In it groups can share their responses to social phenomena, not by organised, cognitive, or primarily verbal responses, but by describing and responding to one another's dreams, and by the exploration of common themes that emerge in a form of collective free association. The primary method is through the creation of a 'matrix', which (somewhat idealistically) is meant to represent a non-individual, trusting, facilitated group atmosphere, able to tolerate uncertainty and non-understanding, reaching, as Lawrence puts it, from the finite to the 'infinite' (Lawrence 2000). Lawrence's 'working hypothesis' is that

> the Social Dreaming matrix, when conducted in an organisation, comes to contain the disowned aspects of the social system, like 'feminine authority'. This is symbolic of all the other disowned aspects of the system. If the

> disowned comes into the matrix, could it not become part of the discourse of an organisation?
>
> *Lawrence (2000, p. 9)*

I shall argue for the RRM as a means of accessing this disowned 'feminine' aspect of interview data, and suggests ways in which researcher and participant, and researchers in relation to transcripts, can begin to create a 'matrix' comparable to that which underpins social dreaming.

Towards the RRM in qualitative research

Let us now examine detailed examples in the literature of 'countertransference' and researcher reflexivity that have contributed to the RRM.

Feelings

Feelings in the researcher inevitably arise in the course of their task, and are sometimes hard to acknowledge: 'whether I wanted them or not, my emotions were phenomenologically present' (Gemignani, 2011, p. 702). Jervis (2011) compares the analytic experience of being overwhelmed with a projective identification (Brenman Pick, 1985), with similar disturbing experiences for researchers using reflexive research methodologies (Lucey, Melody & Walkerdine, 2003).

It has been argued that researchers have resisted viewing their own feelings as influencing, or being relevant to, research outcomes (Lewis, 2008). Emotions will be especially strongly activated in researching sensitive topics, such as interviewing Nazi sympathisers (Marks & Monnich-Marks, 2003) or leaving one's home country, but '[i]f embraced and addressed, the researcher's emotional reactions can be an important source of reflexivity and data' (Gemignani, 2011, p. 701).

Behaviours

Gemignani (2011) speculates that the researcher's *actions* can mirror the psychic experience of the participant. In his work with refugees he distanced himself from painful material, and later thought that in doing so he was '[c]ontributing to the emotional isolation and incommunicability experienced by many trauma survivors' (*ibid.*, p. 701). This illustrates how a behaviour in the researcher can be induced by the unconscious life of the participant, and recalls Sandler's (1976) concept of 'role responsiveness'.

Jervis (2009) highlights this with an example of her conduct with one participant in which she rephrased the participant's word 'terrible' as 'difficult'. For Jervis this represented an 'unconscious collusion in not taking seriously her [the participant's] distressing experience' (*ibid.*, p. 152). Researcher language and rewording is one way in which researchers defensively protect themselves and participants from deeper levels of distress (Devereux, 1967).

Bodily manifestations

Researchers have bodies as well as minds. Some manifestations in the research setting are: 'a fluttery sensation in my chest' (Jervis, 2009, p. 158); 'becoming aware of an attempt to make more eye contact with Joanne [participant]' (*ibid.*); and how other people who had entered the room during the interview were 'largely disregarded by both researcher and participant' (*ibid.*).

These are examples of self-awareness and self-observation which could be seen as useful sources of data.

'Mistakes'

Participants have been described as inducing 'mistakes' in the researcher such as slipping 'out of role'. Strømme et al. illustrate this process in their interview notes:

> I feel that she [the participant] is insecure in her relation to me and that I become unduly avoidant as a response to her uneasiness in the situation.
>
> *Strømme et al. (2010, p. 219)*

Moving away from emotionally charged material on the part of the interviewer could be because 'the interviewer senses that the participant feels vulnerable in front of a critical internalized object projected onto her ... seduced ... into prescribed roles by the participant' (*ibid.*, p. 221).

Here too, from an intersubjective perspective, the avoidance of critical comments, rather than being seen as erroneous research technique, might constitute valuable data in a qualitative inquiry.

Discrepancy of emotional intensity

Projective processes have been described as inducing states of 'emotional mismatch' (Marks & Monnich-Marks, 2003; Lorimer, 2010; Robben, 2012). Robben (2012) describes how researchers (understandably) switched off to strong emotions during interviews with Argentinean war generals who had tortured people. Alternatively Marks & Monnich-Marks (2003) identified a mismatch between the participants' often banal dialogues and the turmoil evoked within the researchers. They interviewed 43 people who had 'agreed to and actively supported Hitler and the Nazi-movement'. Under the subheading of 'countertransference' they state:

> we made, over and over again, the following observations: most of the manifest interview-texts appeared to be relatively banal – compared to the powerful latent (unconscious) emotional message between the lines, occurring during the interviews ... in the course of the interviews we, the interviewers, often felt overrun, bulldozed, emptied, saddened, confused, sickened, abused

> or knocked down. During the nights following an interview we were often haunted by nightmares about war or persecution.
>
> *Marks & Monnich-Marks (2003, no page number, online article)*

Marks & Monnich-Marks (2003) argue that recognising countertransference in the interview setting is difficult:

> such contents are hard to discern in the transcript ... we need to look at ... the message "between the lines", its atmosphere and scenery ... *how* something is being said.
>
> ibid. *(emphasis in original)*

They describe the shame that the interviewers felt when listening to the emotionally disengaged stories of Nazi sympathisers, and describe this as a 'countertransference reaction'.

Summary

Feelings, 'mistakes' and bodily reactions are all unavoidable research experiences, for both researcher and participant, and may be especially prominent and intersubjectively relevant when studying sensitive topics. These transference/countertransference 'markers' include: overpowering, unexpected, anomalous or 'mismatch' feelings; elements of behaviour, e.g. pauses, confused questions and/or responses; difficulties that arise in the researcher (e.g. repetition, asking closed or leading questions) or participant (e.g. incomprehensible or incongruous responses). As we shall see, all of these can be encompassed in the RRM methodology.

RRM: 'sneak preview'

Thus far I have referred to RRM without describing it in detail. The reader will have to wait a little more until the method is elaborated, but here are some observations that show ways in which the RRM both builds on and extends previous work focusing on researcher subjectivity.

We may consider that reverie in the moment of an interview, or when analysing a transcript, is when 'an image presents itself insistently' (Ferro & Nicoli, 2017 p. 73). Such an 'image' may be incongruent, irrelevant-seeming, disturbing, intrusive, 'annoying' (*ibid.*), vague, crisp, motionless, moving, feeling-imbued, related to a bodily sensation etc. Reverie experience arriving into consciousness requires a receptive state of mind, to self, other and felt experience (Ogden, 1996).

Such receptivity may involve focused but non-controlling respectful attention; validation; coupled with, depending on circumstances, support for distress, encouragement of exploration. These guidelines apply both for the researcher's relationship with the participant and his or her internal state.

Reverie is likely confounded if researchers are determined to 'find data', especially those that are pre-formed in their minds. Reverie 'data' is 'hazy' and elusive, and sits uncomfortably with positivist conceptualisations of research even in the qualitative field. Reverie necessitates openness to experience, and the ability to be surprised. As with many qualitative approaches, the research question will usually be found after the research has taken place (Silverman, 2013).

Another element of receptivity to reverie is a quasi-dreamlike state of engagement. This aspect goes beyond some approaches to researcher reflexivity, tapping into feelings that lie on the edge of consciousness. Indeed, Ogden understands reverie as 'preconscious waking dreaming' (Ogden, 2004a, p. 1361). A researcher routinely scanning her/himself and asking 'how am I feeling right now?' may be a start, but may also, to an extent, miss the point. Instead reverie takes 'the most mundane, personal, and private of shapes, often involving the minutiae of everyday life' (Ogden, 1997b, p. 567).

Reverie at first glance may seem to take the interviewer's thoughts away from the participant. Links will have to be made between this apparently 'autistic' aspect of reverie and the interpersonal situation with the participant. A similar paradox applies to silence, which has the potential to be a communicative experience, especially in leaving a space for a reverie image. The researcher's feelings in relation to silence may be the clue to the underlying content, meaning and therefore data. This necessitates an explicit respect for silence, and an acknowledgement that at times research questions may be experienced as directive and contrary to the spirit of reverie.

A final challenge, if appropriate, is for the researcher to volunteer responses to the communicative element which has emanated from a state of reverie. This requires some degree of caution, some degree of bravery, risk and sensitivity, even in data analysis, but especially in face-to-face interviews.

Conclusion

Psychoanalytic ideas offer an alluring field to which a range of qualitative researchers have been drawn. Countertransference-inspired approaches have highlighted the importance of unconscious, 'irrational' and emotional factors in research interviewing. The RRM aims to further develop this approach, showing how reverie, one of the most collaborative and intersubjective of psychoanalytic concepts, can be translated into the research setting. The precepts proposed in this chapter are easier to aspire to than achieve. But before moving to more practical considerations, we need to look at how the RRM stands in the data analysis stage of qualitative research.

5

REFLEXIVITY AND DATA ANALYSIS

'Data' are the raw material of all research, quantitative or qualitative. But what constitutes 'data' is contestable. Scientific advance often occurs through the noticing and exploration of seemingly irrelevant or trivial phenomena – Alexander Fleming's discovery of penicillin is the prototypical example. Thus the concept of data typically implies a clear demarcation between what is considered relevant or important and what is discounted or ignored. How then can we capture, analyse and theorise from the data generated by the researcher and participant's subjectivity – their co-constructed reverie?

This RRM depends on data which is 'emotionally sensed' (Elliott, 2011, p. 3). But can the elusiveness and evanescence of feelings be turned into reliable and reproducible data? Each research interchange contains within it not just its immediate grammatical or procedural meaning, but a web of meanings and associations arising out of the parameters of researcher/participant interaction itself, as well as the personal linguistic and experiential universe of each contributor. 'Interpretation' is unavoidable, arising out of the researcher's impressionistic responses, tempered with implicit or explicit methodological and theoretical assumptions. Even within the 'wild profusion' (Lather, 2006, p. 35) of qualitative methods, guides to data analysis advocate embracing researchers' instincts. This may have a personal theoretical slant: 'try out different theoretical approaches: see what works for you' (Silverman, 2013, p. 58). Qualitative data analysis guidelines 'cannot be reduced to a "cookbook" set of instructions' and instead refer to 'an attitude, an investigation posture with a certain set of goals' (Keen, 1975, p. 41). Thorne (2000, p. 68) reinforces how human interpretation is necessary, and that no computer software package is 'capable of the intellectual and conceptualising processes required to transform data into meaningful findings'.

Hovering uncomfortably around discussions of data analysis is the familiar tension between positivistic approaches and awareness that this may jeopardise the very phenomena it seeks to capture. Rapley (2011, p. 273), tongue in cheek, describes how in qualitative analysis it is:

> *de rigeur* to have some kind of tag. You need the right kind of label in your methods section, ideally one that positions you as competent, so that your work can be nicely categorised.

Qualitative researchers seem intuitively to know that significant data exists at the edge of consciousness and that rich qualitative analysis involves welcoming and using subjectivity, but that this may be at variance with the need for 'objective' methodologies and scientific respectability. Tacit acknowledgement of the importance of subjectivity may explain why data analysis is described as 'mysterious' (Silverman, 2013, p. 56), and often resorts to 'mystical' (Thorne, 2000, p. 68) phrases like 'emerging' and 'sensing'. But data not infrequently is disordered, and analysis more often than not is subjective and interpretative. Language which implies a degree of certainty and scientific accuracy (e.g. 'these themes were extracted from the data') may fail to capture the reality of much qualitative data analysis.

Epistemological perspectives on data analysis of interview transcripts

Categorisation

Strategies such as thematic analysis (Braun & Clarke, 2006) involve categorisation (Polkinghorne, 1995), attempting to bring order into interview transcript analysis (Burnard, 1991, 1994). Categorisation aims to locate or create 'the category of which an item is a member' (Polkinghorne, 1995, p. 10). Categorisation is useful as a means of generating 'knowledge about common patterns and themes within human experience' (Thorne, 2000, p. 69).

Categorisation may bring a feeling of fundamental security through the ordering of experience. Categorisation is the basis of much productive mental activity. 'Mama' might be the first category – a life-saving categorisation! From a research perspective, categorisation may be seen as an essential first step before richer exploration can begin.

But prior categorisation is less suited to data analysis where uncertainty is integral to the topic being studied. This is especially the case when participants are distressed and links to Waddell's (2000, p. 39) description of 'mother's capacity to hold her baby's anxiety and her own, to go on thinking in the face of puzzling and increasingly intense protest and distress'. It is precisely her capacity to avoid jumping in with a 'category' and pseudo-certainty which characterises the reverie-capable mother. The RRM, while ultimately leading to conceptual categorisation, aims at the data collection stage also to hold onto degrees of creative uncertainty. As we shall see later in relation to a specific case ('Tammy',

Chapter 10), by tolerating his own confusion and incomprehension, the data analyst was able, via a reverie image of a stone falling into a well, to establish a theme of being 'dropped' and the relationship between Tammy's depression and her missing, ungrieved father.

Dialectical thinking

Foucault (1972) provided the philosophical foundations for studies which illustrate how power relations manifest themselves in everyday social activity, including discourse itself (Fairclough, 1996). Unequal power relations are particularly prevalent in professional–client interactions such as the doctor/patient relationship (Bunton & Peterson, 1997), and this applies equally to the researcher/participant relationship, structuring their discourse. Dialectical thinking is based on the belief that the structure of discourse is power-related, and therefore that the positions adopted by people in a conversation are frequently, if not invariably, unequal. Dialectical thinking aims to disrupt and challenge what is accepted, and is concerned with the 'social construction of experience' (Kincheloe & McLaren, 2002, p. 88). In the dialectical approach, the 'pristine interpretation' (*ibid.*) is impossible, and no one methodological stance has authority over another. Data analysis should produce rich, socially contextualised interpretations, which take into account the intentions of its producers. The researcher reflects about motivations for undertaking research in the first place, as well as the basis for their interpretations (Basseches, 2005; Srivastava & Hopewood, 2009).

The dialectical approach questions Freud's conception of psychoanalysis as an objective, scientific discipline. However, for Benjamin this is less true of a relational psychoanalysis which prioritises countertransference:

> the theoretical step taken by psychoanalytic thought subsequent to Freud is that the analyst's countertransference recognition – empathy, attunement, and identification with the patient – is as decisive for change as is the modelling of self-knowledge and self-mastery through the interpretation of unconscious forces. It is this step, I suggest, that modifies the link between knowledge and power that critics of psychoanalysis, like Foucault, have seen as indissoluble. It begins to open the possibility of *dissolving* love of authority rather than merely internalizing it.
>
> *Benjamin (1994, p. 543, emphasis added)*

Benjamin here posits a 'pre-dialectical' stage of reverie-driven mother–infant relationship not dominated by power relations. 'Dialectical thinking' may belong to a later stage of development where society and its values begin to instate themselves in familial and intrapsychic worlds. Similarly the RRM also opens the possibility of a 'pre-dialectical' research stage in which the intersubjectivity of the researcher's reverie can access the inner world of the participant.

Phenomenology

Phenomenological research prioritises 'opening ourselves to the phenomenon as a phenomenon' (Keen 1975, p. 38), aiming to shed prejudice, and see the world for what it is. From a RRM perspective, this entails researchers allowing themselves to feel enteroceptive, 'pit-of-the-stomach' sensations, and to focus on seemingly irrelevant, but often salient, visualisations and fantasies in the course of interviews or transcript analysis. A phenomenological guideline would 'sensitize the researcher to a number of issues that need to be addressed in analyzing interview data' in an attempt to understand the 'the world of the unique individual who was interviewed' (Hycner, 1985, pp. 280–281).

Phenomenologists are also wary of categorisation (Thorne, 2000). Phenomenology aims to live with experience itself, and to bring it into focus. Only later will the categorical meanings these images denote be examined. This could be seen as a variant of Freud's 'evenly suspended attention', the stance he advocated for analysts listening to their patient's discourse. Finlay (2009, p. 12) describes how the researcher using Interpretative Phenomenological Analysis (IPA, an approach to qualitative research rooted in phenomenology) should aim to be 'open to the "other", attempting to see the world freshly' through 'disciplined naiveté, bridled dwelling, disinterested attentiveness, and/or the process of retaining an empathic wonderment'.

Phenomenology aims for 'gestalt', i.e. developing a sense for research data and interview scripts in their entirety (Giorgi, 1970). This is achieved through data immersion, for example 'listening to the entire tape several times as well as reading the transcription a number of times' (Hycner, 1985, p. 281).

Phenomenologists emphasise the importance of researcher's subjectivity (e.g. Touroni & Coyle, 2002; Finlay, 2009), and how this will resonate with the research topic under scrutiny. For example, 'in this study, it was hoped that the researchers would be sensitized to different aspects of the data set due to their respective interpretative positions as a heterosexual, female, counselling psychologist and a gay, male, social psychologist, thereby yielding a rich analysis' (Touroni & Coyle, 2002, p. 197).

Critique

These combinations of thematic, dialectical and phenomenological reflections have helped inform the RRM. However an RRM perspective raises some further questions relating to these approaches to data analysis.

1. *Immersion versus first impressions.* There is possibly an overemphasis on the importance of 'data immersion' as a pathway towards understanding. Few would argue against the need for great care and thought in relation to interview data including multiple readings. But it is also possible that the first viewing or hearing of a transcript has a fresh, immediate impact, and this freshness cannot always be recaptured on subsequent exposures.

2. *Participant versus an interactive focus*. Despite Merleau-Ponty's (1962) warning about the limitations of reflectivity, the focus tends to be on *participant* experience rather than a participant–researcher interaction. As Ellenberger (1958, p. 116) puts it, the aim of phenomenological analysis is 'the reconstruction of the inner world of experience of the subject', which may fall short of a full relational understanding.
3. *The researcher's capacity to decide what is and is not relevant*. Here is a key difference. When statements are made 'which are clearly irrelevant to the phenomenon being studied' the typical advice is that they not be recorded (Hycner, 1985, p. 284). These exclusions run counter to a psychoanalytically informed research strategy. The RRM deliberately seeks to tap into seemingly irrelevant but suppressed/disavowed themes.

The RRM draws on the feeling and bodily experience of the researcher as a guide to emotional 'relevance'. Conversely, what might seem like 'model' answer-type responses may be deemed less important, if they fail to arouse the researcher's imagination in the context of the researcher–participant relationship. Reverie provides its own route to truth, no less than, and sometimes in contradiction with, purely logical analysis. Hycner (1985) describes the 'rare and unusual circumstances' where a participant might 'deny what appears to be manifestly in the content of the interview' (p. 292). A reverie approach suggests that discrepancies between the surface and sub-surface meanings of an interview are expectable and ways need to be found to incorporate this into the methodology of the analysis.

Subjectivity in RRM data analysis

Let's move now to a broader discussion of researcher subjectivity and its use in qualitative research. The researcher's subjective responses may tap into interpsychic dynamics, and would in this case 'enrich and deepen' (Kvale, 1999, p. 87) research data.

Cartwright gives an example of how analysing participants' words in isolation (e.g. in an interview transcript) excludes vital elements of data. He describes his feeling of intense fear when a man he was interviewing 'crouched forwards in his chair' (Cartwright, 2004, p. 227). This emotional response was discrepant with the content of the interview in which the participant was talking about his philanthropic deeds. Feeling and bodily states are sources of information in the research process and can be used to contextualise inferences. For Cartwright the participant's bodily posture was vital data which might have been missed in a transcript. Reporting researcher feeling states can enhance reflexive research strategies.

There remains, however, debate in the literature about the extent to which the researcher, modelled on the image of the classical 'intrapsychic' analyst, can remain neutral, or whether, paralleling the 'relational turn' in psychoanalysis (e.g. Mitchell 1990), researcher and participant are inevitably caught up in a mutual, two-way, interpsychic pattern. As we shall see, this dilemma, which has hovered over the whole of the exposition so far, has significant practical consequences.

Some authors (e.g. Jervis, 2009; Strømme et al., 2010) suggest that the researcher's ability to access and think about projected material depends on having completed a psychoanalytic training, or having had personal psychoanalysis. Jervis (2009) suggests that personal analysis provides understanding of one's own defences, and facilitates understanding of what material might be being projected by the patient, and reducing the chances that the therapist's own defences will be ascribed to the patient. According to Strømme and colleagues psychoanalytically informed research will be difficult for an untrained person:

> the psychoanalytically informed research interview requires a researcher with psychoanalytic clinical competence to maximise the potential of this method.
>
> *Strømme et al. (2010, p. 219)*

If a researcher interested in employing psychoanalytic ideas needs to be psychoanalytically treated and trained, this limits its broader research value. Would unanalysed researchers' data amount to 'wild countertransference analysis' (Sandler, 1993, p. 1103)? Psychoanalytic treatment and training is one means of fostering reflexivity, but not the only one (Fromm, 1994). The journey is a personal one for each researcher. The RRM is an attempt to develop methods for using psychoanalytic ideas in qualitative research without the necessity for clinical psychoanalytic training, and find ways in which the method can be taught to fellow researchers.

Morgenroth (2010) distinguishes between countertransference-type reactions that occur in the primary research relationship (e.g. during a research interview) and those that occur in response to text and data interpretation (p. 277). The latter is typically an easier means of accessing such data, since in the heat of the interview the researcher may be too involved to intensively self-reflect. As Devereux (1967, p. 85) puts it:

> the passive spectator role [i.e. someone reading a research interview transcript as opposed to someone actually doing one] does not afford … an opportunity for abreacting anxiety through activity.

Morgenroth argues that the interview data, including unconscious information, captured 'live' in the interview may lie 'housed' in interview transcripts, ready for data analysis:

> as the data are read and discussed by an interpretation panel, so the scene will re- emerge in the feelings of and relations among panel members.
>
> *Morgenroth (2010, p. 277)*

Marks & Monnich-Marks also used a panel to investigate their data, in a process they called 'intervision'. This consisted of group meetings in which interviews were evaluated. During the meetings, the members listened to the interview recording and expressed emotional or physical reactions, fantasies and images about the interview:

> Misinterpretations are possible ... therefore, reactions and observations need to be shared and discussed in group discourses ... in order to find intersubjective consensus.
>
> *Marks & Monnich-Marks (2003)*

This is a valiant attempt, but caution is called for in aiming to reach a 'consensus' in such a process as the essence of some strands of psychic material might produce disagreement (Seitz, 1966)!

Conclusion

This and the previous chapter have examined how qualitative researchers have looked to psychoanalysis when thinking about reflexive practice. Some of these approaches may have imported a classical concept of psychoanalytic 'neutrality', which has largely been superseded in contemporary psychoanalytic thinking, especially in Relational Psychoanalysis (e.g. Mitchell, 1990; Benjamin, 2004; Aron, 1992) and the British Independent Group (Parsons 2007).

Rather than seeing feelings in the researcher in terms of projective identification, with 'useful' and 'interfering' countertransference as separate entities in need of disentanglement, the RRM attempts to develop a more intersubjective understanding, comparable to Ogden's mutually created 'transference-countertransference' (Ogden, 1997c, p. 729). Central to this perspective is an assumption of a 'fallible' (Stolorow, 2003, p. 223) – 'all too human' – researcher. Using this formulation, rather than considering feelings as 'put into' another, they are thought about as filtered through two distinct inner worlds. What results is a situation where

> no thought, feeling or sensation can be considered to be the same as it was or will be outside of the context of the specific (and continually shifting) intersubjectivity created by analyst and analysand.
>
> *Ogden (1994, p. 8)*

In the research setting the feelings of the researcher and participant may be understood as being both inevitably and uniquely linked, while at the same time distinct, as they pass into each individual's subjective experience. Such an approach inevitably brings the researcher's subjectivity more centrally into the picture. The research relationship does not evoke transference and countertransference in the clinical sense. However, when two people come together, the behaviours, words and actions of one of them will inevitably have an effect on the other, at unconscious as well as conscious levels. Before pursuing how this process works itself out in practice, a diversion is needed if we are to establish the ethical and humanistic integrity of the RRM.

6

TOWARDS ETHICAL RESEARCH INTERVIEWING

Becker (1997, p. 151) bemoaned the 'unbelievable sterility of the human sciences' and 'their willingness to manipulate and negate man [sic]'. This can be seen as an outcome of the researcher's psychic defences and hence of the created emotional distance between researcher and researched, and resistance to seeing the research relationship as an emotion-infused relationship, as opposed to instrumentalist data-generation. In other words, this distancing can be viewed as a defensive response, whose function is to protect researchers from the anxieties associated with empathic engagement.

Researchers might convey this stance through their talk with participants:

> 'I want to ask you some questions about …'
> 'Can you help me understand …'
> 'What I'm interested in is …'

Such phrases may appear mundane. However, accompanied with a certain attitude in the researcher, they could contextualise researching as a 'commodity exchange', where the participant, and the interview transcript, become emotionally distant receptacles of information, and the researcher an 'archaeologist' or non-ecologically aware 'mining company' whose job it is to extract information or 'raw material' from participants. The participant is in possession of facts, feelings, attitudes which the researcher wants to access in order to address their research question (as well as, of course, to generate a career, income, a scientific reputation and approval).

As discussed in the previous chapter, the question of motivation forms the basis of a major critique of the research/psychoanalytic comparison (Leider, 1983). In research, the message that the researcher may convey to potential participants is 'I need your help'; in psychoanalysis that is what the patient is asking of the analyst. Apropos the work of Hollway & Jefferson, Frosh & Baraitser (2008) state:

> Vince [the research participant] does not come to them [the researchers] for help – does not feel something is wrong, does not have a sense that the researcher can offer him anything, does not set up that particular transference on which the whole analytic encounter is based. On the contrary, Hollway (who conducted this interview) goes to Vince, wants to interview him, wants to find out something about him, wants to "make sense of him", so the interaction is primarily driven by *her* desire.
>
> *Frosh & Baraitser, (2008, p. 362, emphasis in original)*

In stating that Vince 'does not have a sense that the researcher can offer him anything' the focus is on overt motivations. But there are many subtle reasons why research participants may decide to participate in a study: seeking a chance to talk particularly when the researcher is an unknown, not directly emotionally invested, outsider. There might be the hope that a research interview would provide a fresh perspective on the person's emotional world – a possibility which narrows the gulf between the motivations for research participation and a therapeutic experience. Research interviews of course have the potential to enhance self-understanding, both for researcher and participant.

To the extent that research is about fulfilling a career agenda, or 'getting' participant data only in relation to a predetermined research question, it runs counter to the ethical and pragmatic parameters of reverie described earlier. This recalls Bion's comment, 'if reverie is allowed but not associated with love ... this fact will be communicated' (1962b, p. 37).

Translated onto the research setting, this means that reverie-guided researchers need to attempt to reflect on their motivations and desired outcomes when undertaking a piece of research. Bion's statement also suggests that participants will, consciously or otherwise, pick up on 'research agendas' when these outweigh human concerns. This theme will be explored in more depth in Chapter 9, where the process of switching from a research agenda to speaking from the researcher's feeling state led to unexpected discoveries. For reverie to be accessible, it is imperative that the research relationship be informed by an appropriate ethical stance.

Contemporary views on the research interview see it less as a specialised research tool and more as a set of interactional skills similar to those 'used by all of us all the time in everyday conversations' (Silverman, 2013, p. 164).

The impossibility of interviewer neutrality has been expounded:

> all interviews are active, regardless of how neutral the interviewers and how co- operative the respondents ... no matter how hard interviewers try to restrain their presence in the interview exchange.
>
> *Gubrium & Holstein (2011, p. 150)*

From these perspectives, the research interview is an 'interactional object' (Potter & Hepburn, 2005, p. 281). Language accordingly has a relational feel. Data is no longer 'elicited from' the other, instead it is 'assembled' (Holstein & Gubrium, 2011,

p. 141) in the dyad. Similarly, the interviewer through 'provocations' (Gubrium & Holstein, 2004, p. 150) shapes proceedings, whether he or she wants to or not. However, 'while most researchers acknowledge the interactional character of the interview, the technical literature on interviewing stresses the need to keep that interaction in check (Holstein & Gubrium, 2011, p. 141).

But moving from an explicit participant focus to a more interactional approach is difficult, ethically as well as technically. Hence, a qualitative interview allows: '*the interviewee* the freedom to talk and ascribe meanings' (Noaks & Wincup, 2004, p. 80, emphasis added). This stresses a participant focus, where the interviewer does not assert opinions or make 'any appreciative or critical comments' (Rapley, 2004, p. 21). This is achieved through following up 'on aspects of interviewees' answers' but not straying from what the interviewee is saying (Rapely, 2004, p. 25). Techniques involve unpacking 'key-terms … and while listening, going "mm", "yeah", "right" … alongside nodding, laughing, joking, smiling, frowning' (*ibid.*, pp. 25–26). These are markers which seem to indicate interest in the other, encouragement to continue speaking and also 'affirmations' (although this is left ambiguous – an 'mm' could indicate agreement, but it does not necessarily do so).

In this conception, the interviewer remains a somewhat enigmatic figure for the interviewee. Overtly, interviewers give nothing away about their own opinions. But, as discussed, the perspective of power differentials questions the possibility of research neutrality. For example, interviewing guidelines have been described as:

> replete with masculine metaphors of conquest: probing, directing, questioning, active listening. It is the interviewer who is in control, directing and shaping the course of the conversation.
>
> *Ezzy (2010, p. 164)*

Oakley (1981) describes attempts at objectivity and detachment on the part of the research interviewer as 'morally indefensible' (p. 41); 'personal involvement … is the condition under which people come to know each other and to admit others into their lives' (p. 58). In this spirit, feminist scholars have argued that the interview should become 'communion rather than conquest' (Ezzy, 2010, p. 164), and advocate ethical interviewing as that which attempts to hold in mind the importance of power differentials, and might make attempts to adjust for these, or possibly even comment upon them, which could potentially have an empowering effect on the participant.

Douglas (1985) attempts to move from theory to practice with his technique of 'creative interviewing', which is 'largely based on an understanding of friendly feelings and intimacy, to optimize cooperative, mutual disclosure and a creative search for mutual understanding' (*ibid.*, p. 25). He offers guidelines, which include '[c]ontinuous self-analysis on the part of the interviewer … friendly, caring and adoring feelings … an endearing, wide-eyed sense of wonderment at the mysteries unveiled (*ibid.*, p. 29).

While the aims of fostering wonderment and self-observation are laudable, blanket endorsement of 'caring, adoring' feelings could lead to the denial of other authentic feelings such as hate, boredom, repulsion, sexual arousal etc. In interviews with depressed adolescents, my impression is that a relentlessly positive attitude would harm rather than enhance rapport. Winnicott's (1949) therapeutic guidance again comes to mind, where if 'objective or justified hate' is present the other 'must be able to reach it, else he cannot feel he can reach objective love' (p. 72).

Primacy of the word

In interviewing, the word is sovereign. 'Subordinating' (Stein, 2001, p. 249) other forms of communication and information-gathering to the primacy of the word can be traced to the hierarchical ways in which knowledge is organised and valued in Western society. Words bring order to the chaos of communication. But words may also deceive, and the very order which they bring may be counterproductive, depending on the qualitative researcher's task.

Non-verbal communication has long been of interest in qualitative research (e.g. Ekman & Friesen, 1968; Richmond, McCroskey & Hickson, 1991, Coffey & Atkinson, 1996) but how to access, capture, record and analyse it remain problematic. The issue of interview transcription is crucial. Standard practice encourages the accurate transcription of everything that is spoken, as well as non-verbal sounds such as coughs and hesitations. RRM would add the researcher's sense of the emotional atmosphere, and later the data analyst's waking dream thought or imagistic responses, should these be forthcoming. But such recordings will inevitably be subjective, unlike a cough, which will be heard by all. There is a tension between the desire for objective and replicable qualitative research and the structuration of meaning which identifies salient themes, using intuitive, reverie-like methods to determine what is meaningful.

One phenomenological researcher advocates: 'as much as possible noting significant non-verbal and para-linguistic communications' (Hycner, 1985, p. 280). But how is significance to be determined? And the phrase 'as much as possible' gives a sense of how difficult a task this might become without the researcher using her or his judgement in relation to significance. Ultimately it is a simpler task to objectively record the verbal content of the interview. The RRM attempts to systematise and analyse imagistic non-verbal research data.

Jaspers puts the linguistic problem another way. For conventional research techniques to apply, participants must 'possess the language or written ability and desire to convey their experience' (Jaspers, 1994, p. 311). This brings attention to the danger of researchers 'disregarding what the participants did or could *not* say, or did *not* feel was worth telling' (Gemignani, 2014, p. 133, emphasis added).

Prioritising the verbal content of interviews may mean that researchers distance themselves from emotional communication, conveying the implicit message 'I am primarily interested in what you (and I) *say*'. With this goes the implication: 'I am not (or at best, I am less) interested, in:

how I see you, and how you see me,
how I feel in your presence,
how you speak words,
how you – or I – look bored while we're talking about your family,
how you hold back your tears while you talk about your father's death,
how frustrated I feel with you when you blame your problems on others, etc.'

Interrogatory techniques

While it is well established that effective qualitative interviewing involves more than asking questions, question-and-answer remains the primary dynamic in qualitative inquiry (Britten, 1995). But sometimes questions seem to lead nowhere – the question may fail to produce a meaningful response, or none at all, with the interviewer left feeling baffled and helpless. It is difficult to reconcile an exclusively questioning approach with the need for open and unpressurised space for participants to respond – or not respond – in whichever way they choose. Questions can become a means by which researchers, even if unwittingly, impose agendas on participants, again reinforcing unequal power differentials.

Thus, questions may be experienced by participants (possibly especially vulnerable participants) in ways that the interviewer does not intend. They may be heard as:

1. *Tests of knowledge*. In the study to be described later, one question was reworded from 'having been a participant in the study, what do you think it's all about?' to the more open 'what's it been like being involved in the study?' From the research team's perspective, the aim was to help participants communicate feelings and experiences of being involved in the study, but the reality was that the former wording of the question often brought up a feeling in participants that their knowledge was being tested, and they became uncomfortable. This was in spite of explanations about there not being any 'right or wrong answers' and that this was a chance to think about their experiences in an open way.
2. *Interview as 'attacking'*. If participants are subjected to binary 'doer/done to' thinking (Benjamin, 2004, p. 4), they may experience questions as a form of psychological interrogation or even 'torture'. If this is combined with compliance (see Richards & Schwartz, 2002) the participant may feel attacked by questions, but unable to break out of the interview situation. Participant and researcher may feel chained into the interview schedule, feeling 'we've to get through this'. Each question may be felt as a gruelling task, rather than mutually interesting exploration (cf. Holloway, 1995; Dickson-Swift, 2007). In such circumstances, it becomes especially important that the interviewer uses her

or his sensitivity to gauge how the participant is coping in the moment, and has recourse to change things, possibly by interrupting or ending an interview. Some sense of this 'trapped' feeling, and how it was negotiated, is present in the second extended example presented in Chapter 9.

3. *Conformism versus rebellion.* Although these may appear to be antithetical, both are rooted in 'vertical' power differentials and non-engagement. The interviewer needs to be alert to potential over-compliance, i.e. blind agreement with everything the interviewee says. This may be an indication that the interview is going all too well. Conversely, when questions induce negativity or rebelliousness in the participant, the interviewer may be stimulated into complementary assertiveness or irritation. Closed questioning is particularly susceptible to this form of response, as opposed to more open reflexive or summative remarks.

Questions are just one tool, albeit an essential one, in the researcher's repertoire. There is a need to build on the growing awareness that in research interviewing, feelings states can enhance, modify, contextualise, amplify or diminish the many ways in which both researcher and participant understand words, which are the currency between them.

In addition, as argued earlier, insistence on questioning runs counter to the psychological need for privacy, another cornerstone of reverie. As Ogden states, 'it is as important for a patient to know that he is free to be silent as it is for him to know that he is free to speak' (1996, p. 889). In conducting the RRM a researcher might inform a participant: 'instead of always asking questions, at times I might stay quiet or offer a reflective comment. You are free to respond in any way you choose, which might include not responding at all.' Similarly, an alternative to questioning might be 'thinking aloud' type interventions (Strømme et al., 2010, p. 217). For example, asking things like 'what could have led you to feel like that?' as opposed to 'how did you become depressed?' Clearly, the tone in which this is said is just as important as what is said. The aim is to convey the genuine wonderment felt by the interviewer, if this is felt, rather than convey the sense of having to plough through a set of predetermined questions.

'Interpretation' and 'informed consent'

Melles (2005, p. 21) suggests that research interviewing and counselling skills are comparable: 'establishing rapport, encouraging story telling, using probing questions'. However, for Etchegoyen (1991, p. 417) interventions such as these are 'not part of psychoanalytic technique', because the psychoanalyst's primary role is to interpret. It is difficult to pin down a definition of 'interpretation' in the psychoanalytic literature. Laplanche & Pontalis (1973, p. 227) suggest that 'psycho-analysis itself might be defined in terms of it, as [it is the process of] bringing out the latent meaning of given material'.

Researchers are rightly cautious about 'interpreting' during a research interview. If researchers wish to think about unconscious dynamics, and incorporate these into their interviewing, they must be aware that this process will mobilise anxiety in both participant and researcher, and must be aware that the participant may well *not* be wondering about unconscious motivations.

The question of 'informed consent' in reverie informed research is therefore problematic. The unconscious cannot give consent! A patient can only learn about what psychoanalysis is like by being in psychoanalysis; the patient cannot be fully informed prior to having been in treatment (Hinshelwood, 1997). Similarly, a research participant may be told that their responses will be thought about in terms of unconscious processes, or that interpretation-like responses may be offered, but the only stage at which they would be truly able to 'consent' would be after the event (Rosenblatt, 1995). A participant consenting to such work would only be consenting to their anticipatory fantasies of what it would mean, rather than the reality. A certain leap of faith is required.

Interpreting in a one-off research interview is clearly different from interpreting in the psychoanalytic setting, which usually takes place over a number of years. There is a parallel with a research interview, although of course in the case of treatment, the patient knows this is likely to be the first of many meetings, whereas the research participant knows this will be the first and usually last (although some research designs involve intermittent or follow-up interviews, e.g. life history interviews, Goldman et al., 2003).

Strømme et al. (2010, p. 217) included interpretation-like comments in their research interviews. They interviewed psychotherapy trainees about their experiences of training, with a focus on 'emotional aspects in the participants' experiences'. For example:

INTERVIEWER: I have got one such parallel to what you said about the interview –actually, to be in a situation which is not totally comprehensible. Perhaps that is something you experience as a challenge.

EMILY: Yes ...

ibid. *(p. 223)*

The aim of this interpretation seems to be to imply that the participant was employing similar defensive strategies in the research interview to those in her supervision. The researcher wanted to bring the participant closer to an awareness of her defensive processes. This fits with Weiss's description (1992, p. 292) of interpretation as that which 'helps the patient to gain insight into the maladaptive beliefs and the forbidden goals, thereby facilitating his working to disprove the beliefs and pursue the goals'.

A possible justification for the use of interpretation in the research context is that while it does not aim to produce change or relief of symptoms, it can open up a process of *mutual discovery*. The RRM tries to capitalise on this aspect, not so far removed from some understandings of clinical psychoanalysis. It is relevant that in Stromme et al.'s rather specialised study their participants were psychoanalytic psychotherapy trainees.

Spontaneity and interpretation

Academic psychology has long been influenced by the 'the Cartesian promise of absolute epistemic objectivity' (Bordo, 1987, p. 2). Challenging this, some researchers have attempted to preserve spontaneity of experience (e.g. Munhall & Oiler, 1986) within their repertoire. One technique is to ask participants to describe 'phenomena as fully and deeply as possible, until they have no more to say' (Jaspers, 1994, p. 311). Here participant narratives are 'mined' or 'probed' with further researcher interventions (Gillham, 2005). It is worth noting that this invocation is not 'neutral', as the researcher still has to decide which aspect to probe, and in doing so will thereby betray more of their subjectivity than they may be aware of.

Some have suggested that interpretation in relation to research interviews should be limited to the stage of data analysis, and that recorded interviews will contain deep truths that will be accessed while the researcher is in the process of immersing her or himself in the data. However, an argument for using interpretation-like responses in live research interviews (which as we shall see is part of the RRM repertoire) is that, just as in psychoanalysis, discoveries are often bound up in 'the fleeting and momentary' (Shakow, 1960, p. 90). Paying attention to minutiae can be the most informative. Not responding in the moment to this data might constitute an opportunity lost:

> When there is mutual playing, then interpretation according to accepted psychoanalytic principles can carry the therapeutic work forward. *This playing has to be spontaneous and not compliant or acquiescent.*
>
> *Winnicott (1971, p. 97, emphasis in original)*

The RRM validates researchers' spontaneous responses in and to the fleeting moments of research interviews. These responses emanate not from theory but 'from the groundedness of emotional experience' (Ogden, 1997b, p. 568), and are comparable to ethnographic approaches which rely 'entirely on the spontaneous generation of questions in a natural interaction, typically one that occurs as part of ongoing participant observation fieldwork' (Gall, Gall & Borg, 2003, p. 239).

With these caveats and ethical concerns in mind, let's move now to look at the specific methods and techniques which inform the RRM.

7

THE RRM – THE EMERGENCE OF A NEW APPROACH IN QUALITATIVE RESEARCH

Thus far I have surveyed the theoretical background to using reverie in research, focusing especially on psychoanalytically inspired qualitative research, countertransference and reflexivity. I turn now to an account of my personal journey as a researcher, out of which the RRM evolved, based on three interconnected studies, each with their own methodological strengths and weaknesses.

Methodology and reverie

Reverie is free, spontaneous, unplanned, unexpected, visual rather than verbal, emerging from the preconscious rather than a research protocol. Methodologies which prioritise logical, ordered, procedural descriptions, and which facilitate replicability would therefore view reverie as antithetical to the systematic acquisition of data that is fundamental to this type of scientific enterprise. If it is to be put to creative use, as in *A Midsummer Night's Dream* 'airy nothings' must be 'given a local habitation and a name' (Shakespeare, cited in Schoenfeldt & Schoenfeldt, 2010, p. 64). The first stage of this may be the emergence of an imagic representation of a communicated feeling state. Unstructured reverie may be akin to madness (cf. Milner, 1987; Bollas, 1995; Green, 2012) and unconscious thought is by definition inaccessible to the researcher. The free-floating qualities of reverie must be gathered and tethered. As we have discussed, Heimann (1960, p. 13) questioned the 'un-critical use of countertransference' (i.e. the analyst's feelings), without relating them to the 'actual data in the analytic situation', while Freud (1913, p. 112) described 'spontaneous affect, *but measured out consciously*'. Both imply a tension between the freedom and spontaneity of reverie and the need for it to be held and controlled.

The RRM is not a licence for unbounded freedom (cf. Seale, 2004). Reverie may be born in freedom – but only when securely held by 'method'. 'Method' here is akin to the mother's capacity to contain anxiety – her own and her infant's – and her ability to differentiate them. In research interviews this would mean a tension in which anxiety is neither denied nor allowed to become overwhelming, aiming to provide the safety from which exploration can begin.

RRM practice draws on three basic components: opening oneself to reverie; verbal and theoretical framing and 'binding' of reverie-inspired associations; and negotiating defences. Based on that sequence, RRM comprises a method which entails the following components:

a) focused *attention* on the participant, his/her body posture and gestures as well as words;
b) establishing within the researcher an *inner containing space*; into which
c) *enteroceptive responses* – 'pit of the stomach feelings'; – and
d) *visual imagery* may arise;
e) transforming these sensations into *thoughts*; which, finally, may be
f) verbally *communicable*;
g) which then can be assimilated into a *research hypothesis.*

The three studies

In the chapters which follow I shall give examples of how the RRM works in practice. The first looks at the role of reverie as it spontaneously erupted in the course of 'live' research interviews – somewhat unexpectedly, given that I was at the time following a more conventional research protocol, in spite of my interest in reverie. These experiences provided the germ which grew into the RRM. I unexpectedly found myself experiencing reverie, found this interesting and decided to note and work with it in a more organised way. I then show how RRM can help in studying and analysing interview transcripts. These two studies correspond to two stages of standard qualitative research strategies – 'data collection' (live interviewing) and 'data analysis' (transcript analysis).

Psychoanalytic principles related to RRM

Reverie may be primarily imagistic, but the researcher's capacity to be receptive and responsive to reverie involves a number of additional components. At the risk of some repetition, here are some of the fundamental psychoanalytic principles that inform RRM practice.

Fostering reflexivity. The RRM represents a set of techniques for enabling a specific form of self-reflection in the researcher. Despite significant differences between the clinical and research contexts, if psychoanalysis is seen as one of a range of methods for enhancing self-reflection, research and psychoanalytic aims come closer together.

The unconscious. If people are guided by processes outside of their awareness, conducting and analysing research interviews becomes less about 'fact finding' or establishing 'what really happened' (Stolorow, 2002, p. 335). Instead, it is about building a shared picture between researcher and participant where meaning is personalised, subjective and uniquely formed in the interpersonal field – and often incomplete and inconsistent. It moves away from searching for specific answers to specific research questions (e.g. 'how many weeks after recovery from depression was the participant able to return to school?'), and supports researching in an open-ended way (including acknowledgement of non-verbal or para-verbal communication). A more typical research question which the RRM might illuminate could be 'what understandings of adolescent depression surfaced during this investigation?'

The unconscious 'knows no negatives' (Kestemberg & Zetzel, 1970*, p. 188)***.** Denial can be an assertion, suggesting that the very feeling or thought that is being denied was arising into consciousness, and had to be quickly returned whence it came. For example, an adolescent, discussing his father's abandonment, might say that his dad left the family home when he was a child and therefore his dad is 'meaningless' to him. From a psychoanalytically informed viewpoint this 'meaninglessness' has great meaning. Instead of thinking 'ah this person says it's meaningless, so it must be meaningless' (possibly an example of collusive denial) the RRM researcher will be primed that this area of the participant's life is likely to be connected with feelings of conflict, anxiety and pain, and that this information will be useful for the researcher to *hold in mind* as the interview continues, particularly because the participant's defences around this subject would probably need to be treated with the utmost care.

Psychic defences – in researchers well as participants. Psychic pain is typically managed – repressed, split off, projected, intellectualised – by defence mechanisms (A. Freud, 1937). But the term 'defensiveness' may sound judgemental, especially when defences are conceived on a continuum from 'primitive' to 'mature' (Vaillant, 1977). To conceptualise a 'maturely' defended researcher using reverie to interact with a 'primitively' defended participant takes us back – yet again – to the reinforcement of a relationship of unequal power. But attribution of defensiveness need not necessarily imply denigration. Just as analytic work can be seen as two free-enough minds interacting (including the analyst's as well as the analysand's defensiveness), so the same applies in research interviews. Defences are a reality and can be put to good ethical and research use. For example, the researcher's ongoing sense of the fragility or robustness of the participants' defences will determine how far the researcher goes in exploring a topic.

Transference. If the unconscious is atemporal (Canestri & Fiorini, 2009), earlier residues live on and shape thought and action, including what goes on in research relationships. Awareness of transference, and its 'atemporality', will help the researcher understand the unconscious interaction shaping the data which are presented – and not presented – to him/her in research interviews. The research interview itself can become a source of data 'from the past' under the transference model.

Introspection. In order to use reverie, researchers must be able to look inwardly, to observe their own in-the-moment feelings and fantasies. As Jervis puts it: 'for researchers to really understand respondents' experiences, they must first *feel* them' (Jervis, 2009, pp. 157–158, emphasis in original). The phrasing 'really understand' hints that understanding without feeling-capacity will be insufficient. Researchers must 'feel' respondent's experiences, in the moment-to-moment encounter with the participant or transcript.

Authenticity. Whether self-reflection can be learnt or enhanced now becomes an important question. Reverie is of little use if it emanates from an innate, mystical realm. Although many would argue that reverie makes up but one aspect of psychoanalytic practice, psychoanalytic training suggests the capacity for reverie can indeed be enhanced (but the *selection* of candidates for psychoanalytic trainings presumably suggests that some are seen as having more potential than others). But if reverie is spontaneous and effortless, comparable to a mother's nurturing love for her baby (Bion, 1962b), the idea of 'learning' reverie, in a pedagogic sense, seems bizarre.

> It is not an overstatement to claim that if there is no *feeling with* research participants, the results will be unethical.
>
> *Hollway & Jefferson (2013, p. 164, emphasis added)*

I shall suggest that RRM training can help overcome this paradox, enhancing empathic skills without diminishing their authenticity.

The RRM and parent–infant observation

Candidates involved in many psychoanalytically oriented psychotherapy trainings are required to undertake a parent–infant observation (Bick, 1964), in which the observer visits a family every week for an hour usually for at least a year, and for up to two years. The observer is mostly quiet and passive, absorbing what happens, and then 'writes up' an observational account which is then discussed in a group seminar with other students undertaking their own observations with different families, and a group facilitator. Infant observation is an experience which aims to develop receptive, self-reflexive and empathic capacities which are translatable to the clinical setting (Sternberg, 2005). Thus one aspect of infant observation is fostering in the observer a capacity for self-awareness to the extent that they will be brought in closer contact with their own waking dream thoughts in the presence of the parent and baby. With this grounding, and the commencement of clinical work, the psychoanalytic psychotherapist over an extended period of time may further develop this capacity to the point where the observation of reverie becomes the primary inspiration for the verbal expressions in the moment with the patient, i.e. in reverie-guided interpretation (e.g. Ogden, 1997b, 1997c; Ferro, 2002; Basile, 2006).

With the rise of psychoanalytically inspired research methods it is no coincidence then that recently the relevance of the infant observation model to qualitative research strategies has been explored (e.g. Urwin & Sternberg, 2012; Froggett & Hollway, 2010; Hollway & Froggett, 2012). This method cultivates 'the full emotional attention of the observer … objectivity … in the sense of paying attention to … emotional responses' (Hollway, 2012, p. xiv).

Another way of stating what has been written above is that infant observation is an arena for learning about the usefulness of countertransference reactions (e.g. Sternberg, 2005). Bick (1964), in her manifesto for infant observation in psychoanalytic training, presents a student's observation notes, where the observer's 'tension' is discernible 'between the lines' (ibid., p. 562), for example when an observer attempts to comfort the mother by complimenting her. Waddell emphasises the centrality of self-reflection during parent–infant observation:

> the trainee seeks to observe and inwardly to record not only what is going on in front of his/her eyes, but also what impact this visual record is having on his/her own feelings.
>
> *Waddell (2006, p. 1108)*

Margaret Rustin describes the link to clinical skills, through self-awareness:

> Also vital is a developed sensitivity to emotionality which allows feelings to be recognised by a reflective part of the mind. W. R. Bion wrote of mother's state of reverie in relation to her infant's primitive emotional communications, and something similar is needed both to do a good observation and to become a good clinician. This requires a space in the mind where thoughts can begin to take shape and where confused experiences can be held in an inchoate form until their meaning becomes clearer.
>
> *Rustin (1988, p. 27)*

As Waddell (2006) puts it, the 'psychoanalytic attitude' is encapsulated in the observer who seeks to access 'the potential meaning of the minutiae of moment-by-moment experience both in what was being observed in the other and in what was being observed in the self' (Waddell, 2006, p. 1104).

We have discussed how the theoretical starting point for RRM is Bion's (1962b) theory of reverie. But his mother–infant reverie is dyadic, while infant observation involves *three* subject/objects: parent, child and observer. References to reverie in the infant observation literature largely remain focused on the mother's reverie in relation to her baby. The observer is there in the room, but remains detached. This physical separation extends to a psychological separation when descriptions of the observer's countertransference are either hypotheses about mother–infant processes or those of the observer her/himself.

To illustrate the infant observation situation, here is an example of an extract of an infant observation, where the child was nearly two years old. Abigail is the mother and Alfie her son:

> Up in Abigail's arms, Alfie looks around. Then Alfie says calmly, quietly 'pear'. The observer looks at the kitchen counter. One pear sits there, possibly placed

> there for Alfie to find. Abigail hands it to Alfie. Alfie takes it with both hands. Abigail puts him on the floor and he walks off out of the kitchen with it.
>
> The observer follows tentatively, keeping a distance, not wanting to disturb things. Alfie wants some privacy with the pear. He wanders over to the sofa. He checks on one side of the sofa, then moves to the other side. He squats and moves the pear towards his mouth. Holding it with both hands, he bites into it. The observer sees a white oval of the fleshy part of the pear, where he's bitten away at its dark green skin. He moves the pear in his hands and bites at it again, exposing more of the fleshy part. He chews and makes gentle, determined grunts and breaths. He touches the stalk against his lips, and then the other rough end of the pear which the observer imagines feels sharp against his mouth. The observer now imagines a rougher texture as Alfie bites at a bit near the stalk. The observer becomes aware that Abigail is standing watching too.

In this example, the observer's own experiences interact with Alfie's pear experience. The infant observation technique combines an attempt at a factual, objective description of the mechanics of reality with an imaginative, empathic response, and reflections on both. The observer's experience was stimulated, and partly created, by the intimate proximity of mother and child. The experience of the other is never fully comprehendible. There is always a tension between one's own experience about which, at a phenomenological level, one can hold some certainty, and the 'observing function', where one making inferences about mother and baby's states of mind, and the states of mind which might lie behind these and one's own experiences. From the perspective of 'thirdness', there is an aspect about which one can feel certain (one's own feelings and images), but also another about which there is built-in uncertainty (those of the other). This 'thirdness' has a unique, in the moment, co-constructed, quality – in this case tridaically (mother, infant and observer).

General guidance for receptivity to reverie

Let us return to the psychological conditions needed for reverie to arise and be useful in a research context.

Focus. As will be developed when describing the group form of RRM (Chapter 11), reverie has a meditative aspect. The elements of meditation – sharp focus, single-minded embracing of the present moment and present task – provide preconditions (although no guarantee) for reverie. In RRM interviews, this focal concentration on the present moment may be helpful for both interviewer and participant.

Negative capability. In both interviewing and data analysis, if the aim is to 'extract facts', negative capability is thoroughly disadvantageous. If, on the other hand, when we wish to *feel* something of the experience of the participant (and in the case of transcripts, the participant and the researcher), the capacity to tolerate uncertainty and be open to the unexpected is essential.

Benign scepticism. A balance needs to be struck between interest in how people are – what they say and how we feel with them – and the ability to question and wonder 'what if the opposite were so?' From this stance, a creative conversation can build. This benign scepticism needs to be exercised in the context of safety and a respect for researcher and participant defensive processes. Only then can healthy doubts be entertained.

Holding a hypothesis in mind. Part of this is the 'containment' provided by theory. This must not be a predetermined and rigid preconception, but the recognition that there are patterns and themes to be found among human frustrations, anxieties and life aims, one of the most important of which is a desire for relational self-knowledge.

Setting the scene. From the start of the RRM interview it is important to transmit two features of what is to come – respect for silence, and creative exploration. As suggested in Chapter 6, the reverie researcher will be careful to avoid transmitting the message that the purpose of the interview is only for the participant to 'help' the researcher, since this might impede opportunities for self-discovery. An opening statement might be:[1]

> We have met to think about your experiences of [whatever the research 'topic' may be] but you can say whatever you want, when you feel like it, and I'll respond, if a response comes to me. Sometimes either of us might pause, and be silent for a while, perhaps as we think, and this is fine and valuable too.

Anxiety management. Negotiating interpersonal anxiety is one of the most important ethical aspects of reverie research. It is important to be open to follow-up conversations (e.g. with a phone call), especially if a participant has become distressed. A RRM-type interview is not possible in all cases. Sometimes the formality of the interview situation is particularly anxiety-provoking.

> During an interview with a 15-year-old boy, I stopped making comments and questions which attempted to encourage personal reflection as it became increasingly clear that they were making the boy feel more and more stressed and closed down. Ironically, but true to its paradoxical aspect, *not* having an interview may be precisely the best way to instigate reverie. We stopped the formal interview and I suggested we played a board game while his mum was being interviewed in the next room. During this unrecorded game, his eyes lit up, the mood lightened, he opened up a little about his home life, his cats, his difficulties at school and his absent father.

Conclusion

In this chapter I have tried to illustrate aspects of the RRM 'methodology' – which is, in one sense, also an anti-methodology. Reverie arises in a liminal zone between safety and uncharted waters, between anaesthesia and openness to pain, hypothesising and not-knowing. To apply this uncertainty to the world of research may seem counterintuitive if research seeks out solid 'truths'. However, my contention is that this leads to a reified and reduced vision of human experience. The RRM attempts to capture an essential aspect of experience, opening up a certain type of vision of life and suffering. Part of the inspiration for this vision is the work of the psychoanalyst Thomas Ogden. I now turn to an exposition of his work and how it shaped the emergence of the RRM.

Note

1 In creating this suggestion, I have been influenced by Ogden's description of a possible way of introducing the analytic setting to a new patient. This is in the context of a paper which suggests that outlining the 'fundamental rule' of 'free association', i.e. the imperative for the patient to say whatever comes to her or his head without overly filtering this material, runs counter to his core psychoanalytic principles (Ogden, 1996, p. 890).

8

THOMAS OGDEN AND THE RRM

Let's go back to Karl, with whom we started:

KARL: ... the depression was like a separate feeling to sadness, the sadness would just be like um ... I'm not sure like ... I can't think of an example really but you know not feeling happy just the opposite of happy whereas depression is more like ... I dunno ... sort of ... it's like it goes over all of your feelings as a whole thing and it sort of governs your thoughts as well ...

Which element in a participant's dialogue an interviewer responds to may depend on the atmosphere of interview, and the degree of defensive entrenchment at play, and the degree to which exploration feels manageable. In this instance, we were midway through the interview. Karl was thoughtful and articulate, an aspiring artist, with a rich dream life, both night and day, which he was keen to share with me, in a fascinating, albeit downbeat way. Karl seemed to want to entertain me and capture my interest, while he himself appeared rather bored and detached. I found myself wondering if this dynamic played itself out in other settings. Was he giving me, the 'psychoanalytically informed' researcher, just what I wanted? In the event, I found myself responding:

J: I'm imagining a blanket covering everything ...
K: yeah ... that's some incredi-good example ...

This, for me, was an example of what Ogden writes about in relation to the psychoanalytic situation:

> the analysand's personal psychological space (including his 'dream space') and the analytic space become increasingly convergent and difficult to differentiate.
>
> *Ogden (1996, p. 892)*

The above was an example of the researcher's attempt to make his experience available to the participant, in the service of the research interview itself (cf. Renik, 2004). To further illustrate how this can be accomplished, and bring the RRM to life, in the following chapter I shall present extracts from two interviews with adolescents. In one, a conversational turn, based on the interviewer's reverie, led to an unexpected discovery about the participant's depression. In the second, where the participant was reluctant to talk, the researcher drew on reverie, leading to enhanced rapport, greater spontaneity and the discovery of an 'Oedipal' theme relevant to the origins of depression. But first I want to describe the Ogden-influenced theoretical and clinical background to this project.

Reverie and Thomas Ogden

The work of California-based psychoanalyst Thomas Ogden has been the single biggest influence on RRM. Ogden is a masterful psychoanalytic author, and his corpus represents a body of 'research' of sorts, which captures psychoanalytic experience in a unique way. He is particularly eloquent in his workings around the role of the psychoanalyst's self-analysis. Let's look at his work in some detail.

The psychoanalytic researcher–writer confronts difficulties similar to the clinician wishing to convey their experience of a psychoanalytic session, in that the feeling of psychoanalytic sessions cannot readily be recreated in writing (Ogden, 2005b). The closest one can hope for is a 'poetic' rendering of the experience, hoping to induce visual and corporeal responses in the reader alongside more cognitive or intellectual ones.

Here is Ogden at work (both as a psychoanalyst and a writer):

> My stomach muscles tensed … as I heard the rapid footfalls of Ms. B racing up the stairs leading to my office. It seemed to me that she was desperate not to miss a second of her session. I had felt for some time that the quantity of minutes she spent with me had to substitute for all of the ways in which she felt unable to be present while with me … As she led the way from the waiting room into the consulting room, I could feel in my body the patient's drinking in of every detail of the hallway. I noticed several small flecks of paper from my writing pad on the carpet. I *knew* that the patient was taking them in and hoarding them "inside" of her to silently dissect mentally during and after the session. I felt in a very concrete way that those bits of paper were parts of me that were being taken hostage. (The "fantasies" that I am describing were at this point almost entirely physical sensations as opposed to verbal narratives.).
>
> As Ms. B … lay down on the couch, she arched her back, indicating in an unspoken way that the couch made her back ache. (In the course of the previous months she had complained on several occasions that my couch caused discomfort to her back.) I said that she seemed to be beginning the hour by registering a protest about her feeling that I did not care

> enough about her to provide a comfortable place for her here. (Even as I was speaking these words, I could hear both the chilliness in my voice and the reflexive, canned nature of the interpretation. This was an accusation disguised as an interpretation – I was unintentionally telling Ms. B about my growing frustration, anger, and feelings of inadequacy in relation to our work together.) Ms. B responded to my comment by saying that "that is the way the couch is." (There was a hardness to the fact that the patient said "is" rather than "feels.")
>
> *Ogden (1997b, pp. 572–573, emphasis in original)*

This clinical account contains multiple perceptions of and perspectives on the analyst's reflective self, and the patient–other, including:

- the patient's *movements* ('she arched her back');
- the patient's actual *words* ('the patient said "is" rather than "feels"');
- the *nature and tone* of the patient's words ('there was a hardness' in the way the patient spoke);
- a link to patient's *history* in the analysis ('in the … previous months she had complained … that my couch caused discomfort') (i.e. the 'context', Blass 2013, p. 1129);
- the analyst's *bodily states* ('my stomach muscles tensed');
- the analyst's *fantasies* about the patient ('it seems to me that she was desperate not to miss a second of her session');
- how *bodily responses in the analyst may play into fantasies about the patient* ('I could feel in my body the patient's drinking in of every detail of the hallway');
- the nature of the *analyst's own words* ('I could hear both the chilliness in my voice and the reflexive canned nature of the interpretation');
- the analyst's self-reflection and theories about what he has said, and what he has not said ('I was unintentionally telling Ms. B about my growing frustration, anger, and feelings of inadequacy in relation to our work together').

Again, we see that the setting and circumstances for openness to reverie involve a number of important components. Ogden's psychoanalytic technique incorporates in-the-moment micro-observation and a 'gestalt' consideration of the prevailing patient–analyst intersubjectivity. The more objective observational stance also includes speculative, subjective elements, e.g. the feeling the patient did not want to 'miss a second' of her session. The analyst's communications with the patient are guided by these emotional positions, whether consciously or unconsciously. The analyst's role extends to an awareness of such feelings in the form of more fully elaborated daydream/reveries. Ogden's 'technique' (which, being spontaneous, is also an 'anti-technique') seems to aim to create an internal setting where reverie can flourish, and then, when or if it does, to link these internal experiences to those of the patient.

Here is another of Ogden's clinical excerpts, 'the purloined letter':

> In a recent meeting with Mr L … I found myself looking at an envelope on the table next to my chair in my consulting room … Although the envelope had been in plain view for over a week, until that moment in the meeting I had not noticed that there was a series of vertical lines in the lower right-hand portion of the front of the envelope, markings which seemed to indicate that the letter had been part of a bulk mailing. I was taken aback by a distinct feeling of disappointment: the letter that had arrived in the envelope was from a colleague in Italy, who had written to me about a matter that he felt was delicate and should be kept in strictest confidence between us …
>
> … these ruminations were unpleasantly interrupted by the realisation that my car, which was in a repair shop, would have to be collected before 6:00 p.m., when the shop closed. I would have to be careful to end the last analytic hour of the day at precisely 5:50 p.m. if there were to be any chance at all of my getting to the garage before it closed. In my mind, I had a vivid image of myself standing in front of the closed garage doors with the traffic roaring behind me. I felt an intense helplessness and rage (as well as some self-pity) about the way in which the owner of the garage had shut his doors at precisely 6:00 p.m., despite the fact that I had been a regular customer for years and he knew full well that I would need my car. In this fantasised experience, there was a profound, intense feeling of desolation and isolation, as well as a palpable physical sensation of the hardness of the pavement, the smell of the stench of the exhaust fumes, and the grittiness of the dirty glass garage-door windows.
>
> *Ogden (1994, pp. 5–6)*

Here we get an even more elaborated sense of the interaction between the internal setting, the arousal of reverie and how reverie is processed and thought about by the analyst:

- Letting experience 'wash over' one, expressed by the phrase 'I found myself …' ('I found myself looking at an envelope on the table');
- Comparison of an external object, coloured by the feelings-of-the-moment, with a previous perception ('Although the envelope had been in plain view for over a week, until that moment … I had not noticed that there was a series of vertical lines');
- Observing and linking such 'external' factors with the analyst's feelings ([seeing these lines] producing a 'distinct feeling of disappointment');
- Self-monitoring for 'feelings about feelings': ('I was taken aback by …' [the above feelings]);
- Tapping directly into fantasy images ('I had a vivid image of myself standing in front of the garage doors with the traffic roaring behind me').

All this gives a sense of the reverie method in action. Some critics have worried that self-reference might mean turning away from, rather than relating to, the other: 'the patient's material might get lost when the analyst' is 'so occupied in listening to the activities of his own mind' (Hess, 2000, p. 270). But, continuing the above example, now Ogden provides a relational twist. He views the role of the envelope described above as 'a new subject [the analytic third] … being generated by [between]' the analyst and patient (1994, p. 9). It became a 'new object' when the analyst noticed for the first time the machine markings on the envelope 'in the context of a matrix of meanings having to do with disappointment about the absence of a feeling of being spoken to in a way that felt personal' (*ibid.*). He realised at this moment the extent to which the patient experienced his interpretations as standard, off-the-shelf fare, rather than spontaneous, personal, individualised responses. This in turn opened access to the 'transference' and to the possibility that the patient had similarly experienced maternal care as mechanical and from-the-book, rather than loving and child-affirming, and how at the end of a feed/session the 'garage door' of love and access to 'the breast' was closed abruptly, inflexibly and impersonally. Therefore, Ogden demonstrates in this paper how, by allowing himself to be being temporarily 'lost' in reverie, what was previously inaccessible in the analytic relationship became abundantly available.

Ogdenian research interviewing

Ogden is a master of his craft. But I now want to show how the researcher can aspire to transpose some elements of his psychoanalytic technique into the qualitative research setting. Bion's (1962b, p. 36) pit-of-the-stomach feelings will also occur in response to the emotional entanglement of a qualitative research interview. Converting these feelings into 'verbal narratives' (Ogden, 1997b, p. 572) in the live encounter of the research interview may lend nuance to the conversation. Similarly, applying the same approach to interview transcript analysis might generate novel hypotheses, which can then be tested in further research.

The RRM is a technique relating to research interviews with the emotional communication between researcher and participant at its heart. Antonio Ferro is an Italian psychoanalyst who sees reverie as emanating from the analyst–analysand 'field' (Ferro, 1993, 2009). This is equivalent to the waking dream states discussed earlier: an ever-present component of mental life, potentially accessible to consciousness through reverie.

The reveries to be described in the next chapter were unique creations of the intersubjectivity of the researcher and participant. Before considering them, we need to address the problem of replicability. Another researcher with the same interviewee, or the same researcher with a different interviewee, would have generated different, although possibly related, reveries. Chapter 12 explores this question in greater detail. At this stage it is worth mentioning that the 'site-specific' data which reverie generates have research implications that reach beyond the unique experiences from which they arise.

Ogden's vivid illustrations suggest a number of 'techniques' needed for accessing and using reverie during research interviews:

- *Anticipation.* The interviewer needs to be attuned to the usefulness of reverie, rather than 'pushing away' unexpected thoughts, feelings, images or other manifestations of reverie while conducting interviews.
- *Relaxation of conscious control* – allowing reverie to take its shape or direction naturally. As above, experience in *following* reverie thoughts and feelings will be needed.
- *Overcoming defensiveness.* A key aspect is *tolerance of anxiety*, allowing it to arise, but not to become overwhelmed by it. A partially drifting and de-focused engagement is the ideal here. But interviewers face a number of challenges which may interfere with this process: concentration on aims, such as getting through in the allotted time; prioritising the meaning of the words of the interlocutor at the expense of other factors such as the participant's or the researcher's own bodily responses, or the feelings those words are imbued with; pressure to hold rigidly to the interview frame, and to form over-precise pre-set questions and responses (Wertz, 1986).
- *Reflection.* The researcher will need to reflect on his or her experience of the reverie, paying especial attention to bodily and emotional states.
- *Linking.* This entails thinking about how these states might relate to the participant and/or research topic. As in the psychoanalytic setting, the researcher aims to 'experience and talk with' him or herself about what it feels like to be with the other (Ogden, 1997c, p. 720). Links to the research question or the participant's emotional world may not be immediately apparent. The researcher must withstand the anxiety associated with not understanding. As Ogden puts it: the 'current of reverie is carrying us anywhere that is of any value at all … is usually a retrospective discovery and is almost always unanticipated' (*ibid.*).
- *Utterance.* Finally, the researcher may, if appropriate, put some of his/her reverie responses into words, possibly opening previously unexplored research territory. This last step involves formulating a response arising out of the reverie experience. Ogden describes how in the analytic setting aspects of the waking dream is transmitted to the patient:

> I view reverie as simultaneously a personal/private event and an intersubjective one. As is the case with our other highly personal emotional experiences, we do not often speak with the analysand directly about these experiences but attempt to speak to the analysand *from* what we are thinking and feeling. That is, we attempt to inform what we say by our awareness of and groundedness in our emotional experience with the patient.
>
> *Ogden (1997b, p. 568, emphasis in original)*

Let's turn now from these influences and principles to a detailed example of the RRM in a real-life research setting.

9

THE RRM IN LIVE RESEARCH INTERVIEWING

The research setting in which the RRM developed was a large qualitative study which examined the experiences of depression and recovery in adolescence, by directly interviewing the adolescents themselves. Parents were often invited to take part in separate interviews (see e.g. Midgley et al., 2015, 2016, 2017). This was a qualitative sub-study of a randomized controlled trial which examined the effectiveness of three types of therapeutic intervention on depression (Goodyer et al., 2017). In the two example interviews below, the procedure was as follows. Families were telephoned by a member of the research team. The researcher spoke separately to the adolescent and their parent, explained and responded to questions about the aims of the interview. On the day of the interview, a colleague and the author travelled to the participant's house. While the colleague interviewed the parent, the author interviewed the adolescent in a separate space. Parents were interviewed to gather an alternative perspective on the adolescents' experiences. The interviews had a loose agenda, structured around topics such as experiences of depression and therapy, but also aimed to enable participants to express themselves (which was often a struggle with depressed adolescents). This latter aim afforded exploration of the reverie interviewing method. Interviews were recorded on a Dictaphone, and each lasted about an hour. They had consented to take part in the study. Identifying details, venues and clinical aspects have been disguised. Two examples are presented, Ann and Lizzy (pseudonyms). Moments of reverie are presented in square brackets; additional information such as intonation in round brackets; and comments in italics.

Reverie in the interviews is initially accessible through awareness of general feeling states (e.g. uncomfortable, claustrophobic feelings; as above, 'in the pit of the stomach' feelings), which may then produce an image. The reverie described in the research encounters below were, at the time of the meeting, 'almost entirely physical sensations as opposed to verbal narratives' (Ogden, 1997b, p. 572). Converting these feeling states into written formulations came about during the post-interview phase where the researcher 'felt around' the encounter.

Interview 1: Ann, the 'weird birth'

As the researchers arrived, builders were outside the house, in sight and earshot, at times. Ladders and papers were strewn about. The interview took place in the dining room, which opened onto the sitting room where a restless dog was caged. Ann and her Mum (being interviewed upstairs) negotiated the dog's care at times.

Ann seemed energetically anxious, with staccato speech patterns flashing from idea to idea. Often, she said 'like', and spoke with a rising inflexion.

This is a 5-minute segment from the middle section of the interview:

ANN: … like I'm quite confident and stuff and like I'm quite happy like probably underneath all this stuff there'd probably be like a trigger like my (*background talking*), d'you know what I mean? (*Voice trailing off in a distracted way*) I think I've always had a little bit of something like depression in me … that can get triggered … like I think it's inevitable really.

[Baby Ann, and comparing her experience to that of the dog in the house. 'Something … underneath' may lead to thoughts about her babyhood. Interviewer feeling distracted and overwhelmed, and wishing for more space to think].

J: You've put an image in mind of you seeing depression as a little thing that's lurking inside you.

The phrase 'little thing' could convey the baby reverie, and the word 'lurking' may imply neglect.

A: yeah, I think it is you know … it's like a tumour (*she laughs*) just in there … it's like I think it's like a … a birthmark, but not really a birthmark … a mark that will last a few years that will probably stay with me forever like I'll always remember it and it always comes back to me (*others talking in the background*).

[A tumour, hidden beneath the skin, then surfacing and visible as a birthmark]

(*Dog barking. Shouting to her mum about the dog*) I'll put him outside, it's fine. (*To dog*) Come on! Out, ok! (*Door slams*). (*To me*) He's gone now! (*Both laugh gently*).

J: You were saying depression's a bit like a … birthmark.

A: Birthmark's not a great word like, like it's always gunna be a scar it's always gunna be with me but like … I will always remember it and I can always be affected by it.

[Imagining her birth itself as scarring]

A: Like if you look at your scar it's like you go back to it, like you can feel like … you can feel the pain or whatever and then it can like – d'you know what I mean? I'm not explaining it well but I'm just being like poetic (*earlier she spoke about enjoying poetry*) …

J: And this may sound like a funny question but … do you know what your birth was like?

Perhaps unconsciously responding to Ann's repeated use of the word 'like', but taking it more literally. I see surprise cross Ann's face and she responds.

A: Oh, I was um, C-section and I was like sitting up, I was breech so ... sort of like that. Is that like – does that –

J: (*interrupting*) No it was just ... it just came to my mind 'cos you said birthmark ... I dunno why.

She is able to respond to the question and it sounded like a traumatic birth. An area of interest is opened – and possibly not explored as fully as it could have been – impeded by my protective, and perhaps defensive, interruption.

A: It is kind of a weird birth to be honest like it's not natural so I 'spose, I dunno, but yeah ... that's like also another thing – I see – 'cos I study psychology as well so I see it in a very – I've kind of pieced myself apart while I was doing it.

Discussion of the interview with Ann

Before the word 'birthmark' was spoken, reverie brought 'baby Ann' into the interviewer's mind. She had described something 'underneath' being the 'trigger' of depression, the 'little thing', 'lurking inside her'. She then described depression as a 'tumour' and a 'birthmark'. These were consistent with the sinister reverie, which later led to the question of her birth, which was 'weird'.

The first reverie experience may have been evoked by perceptions about the environment (disruption and caged dog), the interviewee's 'style' (Ann's enthusiasm) and the interviewer's inner state (wanting a quiet moment). The dog-distracted images stimulated thoughts of Ann's babyhood (dog-dependency-baby-distraction – what is being distracted from? – something painful). Next, her comparing depression to a '*birth*mark' contributed to the question about her birth.

The above gives a sense of the interview as a mutual creation, moderated by reverie, akin to Winnicott's (1965a, 1965b) 'squiggle game'. Ann offers a vaguely ominous picture: 'something', 'underneath', 'always ... in me'. Reverie locates and verbalises it – 'lurking', i.e. invisible, or shadily visible, in the pit of her self. In the next brushstroke, the figure becomes tumorous, and lodged. Possibly to escape from anxiety, the tumour now becomes a 'birthmark', scarring but benign. Having been 'drawn', the birthmark is quickly 'scribbled out' ('not a birthmark'), but the scribbled mark remains 'on the page' in our minds. The next move is more verbal, less reverie based, pointing to the thought, circling it – effectively 'saying' – 'it may have been scribbled over but let's see if we can have another look'. Ann looked surprised; the drawing becomes 'factual', anatomical: her breech birth, baby-Ann starved of oxygen and in danger, but having survived to communicate this.

The question about Ann's birth was a departure from Ann's conscious communication. Whether this departure was helpful or unhelpful is open to question. On the 'helpful' side, a conventional research interview strategy might have encouraged the researcher – in response to hearing 'I've always had a bit of depression in me' – to say 'can you say more about that' (see the second example below where this is done, unproductively), which, while unexceptionable, might also have been a defensive avoidance of both interviewer and interviewee's approach/avoidance oscillation with the anxiety-laden topic of birth and permanent psychological scarring. The word 'birthmark' could be viewed as a 'switch word' (Freud, 1901, p. 274), and an entrée into the unconscious and live themes for Ann. On the other hand, perhaps this was an interviewer at the mercy of interfering countertransference (Heimann, 1950), where his fantasies and associations had little relevance to what Ann was communicating. Ann was engrossed in wondering about how depression may have affected her in the future and, based on a reverie experience from several moments earlier in the interview, the interviewer abruptly moved the focus to the past. The reverie-guided question could have been viewed as impoverishing the interview, a 'foreclosure of meaning' (Cooper, 1993, p. 95) which prematurely directed Ann's own imaginative exploration.

Whether viewed as useful or not, reverie was undoubtedly drawn on in a rather direct and clumsy way. Researchers inexperienced in using reverie need to be wary about premature or too specific verbal expressions of reverie.

Interview 2: Lizzy, 'no' and 'yeah'

Lizzy let us in and went and sat still on the sofa. We waited for quarter of an hour for her mother to come home from work. My colleague and I made some attempts to engage Lizzy but to little avail. Had Lizzy been pressed to do the interview by a parent? I felt daunted and protective, thinking she might be nervous about being alone with us, unknown people. Once her mother arrived, my colleague went off with her to an adjacent room, separated by a thin door through which the murmurs of their conversation were audible. Perhaps encouraged by this maintained link, I asked to sit on the large sofa with Lizzy for our interview. She had been speaking so quietly and I worried I wouldn't hear. She said 'OK'.

I noticed myself speaking cautiously and quietly. Soon I felt uncomfortable and thought that Lizzy probably wouldn't have been able to tell me if she hadn't felt OK about me moving closer to her on the sofa. Lizzy sat facing forward, not looking in my direction. I had little sense of her face or expression, which her hair obscured. (I am partly aware of these things retrospectively through comparing how I saw her in the moment of meeting, contrasting with her as we were about to leave, when I remember her as rosy-cheeked and smiling, standing next to her mum).

The interview began:

J: Thinking back to when you were first referred to (*name of clinic*), what sorts of difficulties were you going through?

L: I went the doctor's, my GP said that I … um … I dunno, that I … was feeling low and I was tired a lot and sleeping a lot and … anxious … and then he referred me to (*clinic*) … Yup.

J: Ok, so you were feeling tired a lot …

L: Yup

J: And anxious too ...

L: Yup

J: Could you say a bit more about those anxious feelings?

I notice the tentative, cautious tone. So many questions!

L: Umm ... I stopped going to school and going and out with my friends and ... Yeah.

[Discomfort. Questions failing. Finality in the 'yup's and 'yeah's, closing doors]

Lizzy then told me stiltedly that her anxious feelings had started the previous autumn and seemed to be brought on by having to go to school, I ask:

J: Had something happened at school?

[Spoken in a particularly weak voice, the word 'school' trailing off, as though I'm scared I'll enrage her, or I'm ashamed of the intrusion]

L: No

[I hear the 'no' as weary, condescending – a response to my pathetic vocalisation, almost as though there was an upper hand to be gained and Lizzy had done so. It conveyed a feeling of 'again, you're asking me to tell you about how difficult feelings emerged. I won't!' The 'no' was also said almost instantly and felt stabbing, and I think she must have been asked this question before]

J: So you know ... have you got any theories about what was going on?

I press on in spite of inner discomfort.

L: No

J: I guess it's hard to know sometimes. Sometimes we just start to feel things and we don't know why we feel them.

The phrase – 'you know' – could be seen as descriptive, responding to all the 'no'-ing! The latter response may have been an attempt at reassurance – that it was alright not to know (and hopefully that it would also be alright to not 'no'/know, i.e. to speculate and explore). Lizzy seemed fearfully closed off from the conversation.

J: Is the question of how those feelings developed something you've thought about?

After attempting to acknowledge her feelings, this tacitly reverts to script in questioning her about meaning. With hindsight, it seems obvious that this dynamic was partly what had led to such a stilted communication. But Lizzy responds:

L: Yeah

Now Lizzy effectively tells me 'yes, I've thought about it, but that doesn't mean I'll tell you about those thoughts'. She has stopped 'no'-ing at last, although her 'yeah' here is a sort of 'no'!

[Lizzy in her therapy. She's talking freely with her therapist in marked contrast to how she is with me]

Lizzy spoke about the improvements she'd felt that therapy had brought to her life. She said that these days her anxiety was based on 'normal' things like exam stress and fights with friends. I asked her whether the anxiety she used to feel *hadn't* felt normal. She replied that it hadn't. I asked what the difference was between the 'normal' and the 'not normal' anxious feelings.

L: Well I didn't have any reason to be anxious, like there was nothing at school to make me anxious.

(*Ten seconds pass in quiet*)

J: I have a … sense while I'm talking to you that … it's like you've been asked all these questions hundreds of times before.
L: Yup (*she smiles; the first time I've seen her smile*)
J: (*gentle laugh*)

Relief seeing her smile for a moment. A breakthrough?

[Imagining a similar sequence playing out with her therapist. Now seeing a warm relationship. She and her therapist are sharing a joke about her involvement in the research project, all the forms she's filled in and generic questions she has been asked about depression]

Until this point 'reverie interviewing' had entailed micro-observations of words and bodily changes. Then the interview dynamic changed. Lizzy became more relaxed and spontaneous, and less hostile. She spoke about the moment her therapist told her she was pregnant:

L: But (*name of therapist*) is leaving anyway in November for maternity leave so we can't continue longer than that.
J: She was going to have a baby. At what point in the therapy did you realise that?
L: Only like a month ago, less than that, about 3 weeks ago.
J: Do you remember what you felt?
L: Well it was after we'd organised all the sessions and she was just (*clears throat*), she was like asking how it was at the beginning, and then she was like 'I've got some news, I'm having a baby.'

Lizzy says her therapist's phrase very quickly: is there no time to work out what she felt? Questions are no longer tortuous, but useful.

J: Was it a bit of a shock?
L: No … I knew she was gunna have a baby.
[Affection and envy in her voice, I notice Lizzy is also able to refute and correct my question. Both this emotion and this correction would have been unthinkable earlier. The correction fills the space with something – like a baby growing – whereas before there was emptiness, a vacuum, rather than a space open to meaning (or pregnancy!), in the refutation]
J: How did you know?
L: I just knew! (*Laughs*)
J: Do you remember at what point you knew?

L: No. I just knew, and she, she was like 'I've got some news'. And I was like 'she's having a baby'.

J: Had you seen her bump?

L: No, she doesn't really have a bump even now (*sharp intake of breath, as though she's just remembered something*) ... oh she kept putting her hands over her stomach.

J: So you'd noticed that.

L: Yeah.

J: Did she say anything else about having a baby?

L: We've spoken about the baby a bit.

J: What was that like for you?

L: Good.

> *The interview seems now to have regressed to less connected relating. Asking 'what was that like for you?' was more of a classic, neutral 'interviewer stance' and possibly became too persecutory, as though I lost my ability to trust reverie as a gauge of what it was like for her and needed to ask directly.*

Discussion of the interview with Lizzy

Before the interview started I had felt protective. As it began, I felt excluded. Through the emotional charge of her words, Lizzy was effectively communicating 'I won't engage with you like this', offering a challenge to try something different. After her repeated 'no's, a comment was offered ('sometimes it's hard to know'). In response to the next question about whether she had thought about the origins of her depression she said 'yeah'; this led to a reverie in which I imagined her with her therapist, while I remained excluded. Lizzy still responded with one word, but her affirmation stimulated 'seeing' her in therapy. Thus, the 'yeah' seemed to induce a 'piecing together' image, akin to the fantasy image summarised above in Ogden's reverie (although far less elaborately visualised than in his examples). This suggests three kinds of reverie all of which were in play in the interview: the *autistic* model of reverie, which is 'no' related: a *compensatory* reverie to mitigate the loneliness of rejection and exclusion; and a *relational* reverie stimulated by 'yeah', which is an invitation into a jointly peopled field.

After imagining Lizzy in lively conversation with her therapist, where they joked about regimented research meetings, such as the one we were in the midst of, it was wondered if she had been asked these questions 'hundreds of times before'. At this point Lizzy became enlivened. She engaged somewhat playfully, conveying affection for her therapist, as well as *her* painful experience of exclusion in the story of her therapist's pregnancy (which became both a 'yeah' and a 'no'). This reverie of exclusion from the therapeutic couple on the part of the researcher chimed with Lizzy's response to her therapist's pregnancy. This in turn pointed to a link between her depression and a comparable Oedipal exclusion. This had possibly been present in the interview from the start when Lizzy was alone, waiting for/excluded from her mother, both inviting me to protect her and keeping me at a distance, for fear that I too would leave her, pregnant with my research findings, but leaving her empty and abandoned. The appreciation of this seemed to lead to her softening. By the moment of parting, as she stood beaming next to her mother, I wondered if she felt she had fought through something difficult but valuable.

So we see how a reverie-guided intervention brought what would otherwise have been a flat, somewhat depersonalised interview to life, and led on to interesting material about the therapist's pregnancy and its unconscious resonance for the interviewee. It could however be argued that psychoanalytically informed reverie was not relevant in the above interview. The situation of an interviewer attempting to interact with an unresponsive interviewee is not uncommon in qualitative interviewing. It is in just such tricky situations where skilled qualitative interviewers may turn to their subjectivity as a source of inspiration, and this is not dependent on psychoanalytic knowledge or expertise. Against that there is a case that the developmental ramifications of Lizzy's depression were exposed via this reverie-inspired intervention, going beyond merely 'unsticking' a rather stilted interview.

Discussion

The following section outlines the values of reverie-informed research interviewing, and responds to potential criticisms. It is suggested that using reverie-guided language deepens research interviews without necessarily distorting them, and yields relevant data on the research topic that would otherwise remain unearthed.

Language and reverie interviewing

In conventional interviewing participants are typically invited to give verbal descriptions of emotional states. But from a psychoanalytic perspective language may be as defensive as it is revealing. But words are perhaps better seen as outcomes of emotional states, rather than accurate representations of emotions. Reverie sits ambiguously in relation to language: ultimately revealing itself through language, while at the same time deriving from 'pre-linguistic' phenomena such as bodily sensations and visual imagery. It may either be the emotional tone ('the way' of speaking being just as important as the content, Ogden, 1997a, p. 1) that triggers reverie, as with Lizzy, or the use of jarring, anomalous words, such as when Ann speaks of a 'tumour' and 'piecing herself apart'. In the interview with Ann, the communication explored links between the verbal and imagistic connections along a chain of meanings: depression/'tumour'/birthmark/Caesarean birth. Metaphor – etymologically a 'carrying across' – entails finding similarities in apparently dissimilar phenomena. Feeling at home with reverie helps therapists and researchers navigate these metaphorical waters and backwaters. Lizzy, by contrast, used language more concretely. Here the interviewer him or herself has to be the source of the metaphor: in this case finding the 'metaphorical' parallel between Lizzy in therapy with her pregnant therapist, and Lizzy in the room with the researcher.

The potential 'research yield' of reverie-informed interviews

Both interviews identified significant themes relevant to adolescent depression. In Ann's case a developmental rather than purely symptomatic model is suggested, linking a difficult birth, with possible ramifications for her early relational experience, with a sense of 'scarred' or defective self – rendering her vulnerable to depression. In Lizzy's case depression becomes 'triadic' in that, using an Oedipal model, there is always an excluded third party, whether this be the researcher or Lizzy and her mother, Lizzy herself and the pregnant therapist. Her capacity to work through this with her therapist, and therefore to become more resilient when feeling excluded by her peers, comes to the surface via a simple reverie-driven attempt on the part of the interviewer to overcome *his* sense of exclusion.

Despite these advantages, a number of criticisms can be levelled against the reverie method.

Critique 1: A research interview is not a clinical session, and the participant consents to the former, not the latter. Offering interpretation-like interventions in interviews raises ethical questions.

As mentioned, a reverie-driven research interview may well develop a 'clinical' – i.e. confidential, emotionally live – atmosphere. Indeed, the more clinical-seeming the interview, perhaps the more successful it will be, in that it will have facilitated hitherto latent emotional expression. This argument can be viewed as a reversal of Freud's view that every psychoanalysis was a species of research (Freud, 1912) – i.e. every research interview, if reverie-informed, can also be 'therapeutic'.

Furthermore, the reverie-informed interview method bridges the research/therapy gap yet further in setting aside formalised research questions and agendas, because this will interfere with the aim of eliciting spontaneous conversation. It might be argued that the interviews in this study were particularly 'clinical' for a number of non-generalisable reasons: the participants had had therapy; the interviews specifically aimed to elicit stories about the experience of depression; the interviewer had supervision from psychoanalytically oriented clinicians.

The critique here is that the interviewer in these examples strayed from his researcher role to that of a therapist. Asking about Ann's birth was, from this point of view, when the research stance was abandoned for a clinical approach, and the birthmark question was an implicit – and unwarranted – interpretation about the circumstances of Ann's birth. The notion of an interpretation occurring in such a setting jars because – in spite of Freud and his reversal – there are enduring differences:

a) Aims: the aim of eliciting spontaneous conversation is only one strand of psychoanalysis, which also may aim to alleviate psychic suffering of patients. Qualitative research's aims are different, i.e. information gathering. This difference lessens if the reverie research method, as is claimed here, enhances the garnering of relevant information.

b) Continuity: psychoanalysis takes place over a number of years and between four or five times a week, while qualitative research interviews are typically one-off meetings. But this quantitative measure does not stand up, given that even a single session can be psychoanalytically informed.
c) Privacy: apart from cases such as potential violence or child protection, psychoanalysis is inherently a private matter, patients have the final say whether data from their analysis may be shared or published. In the context of 'consent' the same applies in research but there is an understanding from the outset that the aim is dissemination. This means that the endeavours will likely be entered into in different states of mind.
d) Training: The psychoanalyst undergoes a rigorous training involving their own psychoanalysis, supervised clinical work and theoretical input over a number of years. Most qualitative researchers have not undergone such a training. This raises the danger of 'wild' or even unethical reverie.

The case of Ann illustrates how this method necessitates a skilled interviewer who judges how a participant may assimilate a reverie-informed communication. Asking Ann about her birth, when she was not (consciously) thinking of it involved some risk. Responding by saying: 'when you said "birthmark", I wondered about your own birth ...' may have been experienced less joltingly, and would have given Ann more of a chance to work out how safe she felt before responding, or not responding. *Critique 2: This approach is not useful for* researchers *because it is not scientific; a key problem being the lack of replicability.*

Clearly, this approach is located within an alternative, non-positivist epistemological tradition, with its own conceptions of scientific validity and replicability (Parker, 1998). This study has not been able to fully address the replicability issue. A later chapter explores this further, in which several researchers were invited to independently examine the same section of interview transcript. It seemed that there is in fact often convergence of themes in response to the same section of interview transcript, notwithstanding that the specific imagery of the reverie remained personal. The question remains to what extent reverie experienced by a research interviewer is connected to psychic communications between interviewer and participant, and to what extent it is an isolated (and therefore potentially isolating) experience generated in the mind of the researcher. The relational perspective implicit here views reverie as essentially co-created, and that, while coloured by the interviewer's preoccupations, it provides a window into the feelings, meanings and conflicts of the interviewee. Reverie can therefore yield relevant information about the research topic inaccessible to standard interview methodology.

Conclusions: 'the core theme'

Reverie-informed interviews are intersubjective dialogues in which data arises as much in the responsive mind of the interviewer as it does in the interchange of words. Once openness to reverie is included in the qualitative research repertoire, reverie-influenced 'leading' becomes a useful and usable tool in research interviewing. This chapter illustrates how an awareness of reverie can serve at least two purposes in research interviews. First, researchers' emotional reactions, bodily sensations and mental images, if incorporated into communication, enhance rapport-building, and therefore alter the texture of interview material.

Second, reverie can be informative for the research process itself. In both interviews, reverie which might have seemed irrelevant unearthed stories of adolescent depression – in one case birth trauma and a feeling of 'weirdness' (cf. Blatt, 2008), in the other Oedipal exclusion (Taylor, 2009). These findings can be turned into more formal hypotheses as well as potentially useful pointers for psychotherapists. These will centre around a 'core theme' which encapsulates the essence of the research question, emerging from reverie-based phenomenology, but with more general implications.

Ann's case suggests that there is a retrospective elaboration of a 'depressive life story', starting with or before birth; this makes meaning out of inchoate mental pain and so provides a measure of reassurance, making her depression more manageable, meaningful and less 'lurking'. A more negative dynamic, and one which is relevant to depressive relapse, generates a sense of an inescapable fate; distraction – which a conventional interview might represent – takes the depressive away from these feelings, but if not challenged they are likely to return. In Lizzy's case, her depression is linked with a sense of abandonment, with developmental experiences in which feelings of exclusion predominate over connection and communication. Acknowledging that interpersonal gulf helps relieve depressive feelings, and establishes connection.

Reverie brings closer to consciousness the intersubjective emotional potential which lies at the heart of – but is often evaded in – qualitative interviews. There are various overall principles which can guide reverie informed interviewing: silence is potentially communicative and valuable; questions are but one of several ways in which communication can be facilitated; an interview is a unique event with an unique individual and thus, although the research protocols provide a useful overall structure, research questions, especially in exploratory and early-stage research, will often become clearer only *after* the interview.

Birksted-Breen (2012, p. 819) argues that 'in order to be psychoanalysis, the "here and now" technical approach requires … "reverie" … without this … attention we have two people in a room but not psychoanalysis'. Without reverie, qualitative research might be two participants filling in forms, or staying near the surface, but missing the opportunity to embark on productive journeying into the unknown.

This study represented my first experiences of reverie in a research context. The next chapter shows how the RRM begins to be systematised, and how it can also be applied to interview transcripts.

10

RRM AND INTERVIEW TRANSCRIPT ANALYSIS

> A sandcastle washed away by the sea. Clumps in the sand where it once stood. Soon, even these will be gone, wiped out by the waves, and flat sand will be left. *I* (Mum) know what used to be there, but others may not.

Following the 'data collection' of research interviews, the next step in most qualitative research strategies is to convert the recorded words of an interview into text, to create a 'script' which can then be subjected to the process of data analysis. This chapter explores how the RRM can be used at this stage of researching.

The above example of reverie (to which I return below) came to mind in response to a two-person interview dialogue recorded in the form of a transcript. Text can create a feeling-imbued imaginative experience for the reader. Freud described reading novels as having the potential 'to make such an impression ... and to arouse in us emotions of which, perhaps, we had not even thought ourselves capable' (1908, p. 143). Himes poses the question:

> Where does the meaning of the text lie? In the hands of the original speakers, or by the experience of the reader, or in the relationship between the speakers and the reader?
>
> *Himes (2001, pp. 335–336)*

Psychoanalytic data analysis

There is a small literature on psychoanalytically inspired approaches to data analysis (e.g. Whitehouse-Hart, 2012). Some psychoanalytic authors have compared reverie in response to texts to reverie in the clinic in relation to patients (Paikin, 1995;

Gliserman, 1996; Hurst, 1998; Meltzer, 2003). As mentioned, Ogden, (1997c, 1999, 2001, 2004a) is prominent among these.

The technical distinction between reverie generated while in the presence of another person, as opposed to while reading a text, bears consideration. It might feel for the reader that we are changing perspective – quite abruptly – from the live interviewing encounter into a different situation, in analysing an interview script, which is several steps removed from the interview itself. Nevertheless, in both situations, there is a researcher with the potential to foster an inner space where reverie may flourish. The interview transcript is an emotional interchange captured in text, playing itself out on the page. While the live research interview may have more in common with a psychoanalytic session, the data analyst of an interview script may assume a role closer to that of the supervisor of a piece of psychoanalytic work who might experience reverie, while studying the process notes of the supervisee.

In terms of practical realities for reverie generation, the emotional immediacy of the live interview has advantages and disadvantages. While studying an interview script, the researcher has the luxuries of time and distance. Studying a script can happen in relative tranquillity – in external reality – which may provide the researcher with more internal space to experience (rather than need to defend against, as is often the case live in the encounter) the potential confusion and emotional turmoil of the interchange. Transcript analysis may also be akin to what Ogden describes as 'listening' (Ogden, 1997d, p. 619) in relation to poetry, where the reader's 'ear' (standing for a receptor organ for emotional experience) is activated. However, the studying of a script is potentially open to a more 'wild' type of analysis, as there does not exist the possibility to explore the relevance of a reverie experience based on the prevailing and in-the-moment emotional atmosphere, as exemplified in the above chapter. It is true that much, but not all, is lost from the original encounter when it is reduced to a verbal interchange and read. Thus, while this chapter will lay the groundwork for the idea of an individual researcher using reverie in relation to interview transcripts, subsequent chapters examine what happens when multiple researchers independently study the same transcript, using RRM, before these responses are compared. This is an essential step in increasing the reliability of RRM-derived data analysis.

Retaining openness to uncertainty while seeking valid research 'findings' remains problematic. Thus Ogden is suspicious of attempts to make Bion's work more accessible, if this 'is to diminish, if not completely ablate, the impact of Bion's radical reconfiguration of many of the fundamental tenets of psychoanalytic theory and technique' (2004b, p. 286).

Ogden's caution about taming Bion's radicalism can be compared with research techniques in which the lived life of the individual participant is necessarily assigned to predetermined broad-brush categories, when cross-comparing or distilling themes across a number of research participants. In doing so, the initial meaning, often complex, chaotic and confusing – but perhaps containing the very 'data' which is sought – may be lost. With the above caveat in mind, let's look at how the RRM tries to circumvent this problem.

Interview dialogues may at times be chaotic, unintelligible or sparse. In the examples below, this was at times the case in encounters with adolescents who had been asked to take part in reflexive, open-ended interviews. This is unsurprising given that adolescence itself, and especially in depression, may in some circumstances be characterised by introspection, non-responsiveness, blocked reflexivity and struggles to meaningfully link with another person who may seem to be in a 'parental' position of authority (Midgley et al., 2015). In relation to clinical psychoanalysis, Rosenfeld (1952, p. 117) notes that when the patient has 'great verbal difficulties' the 'unconscious intuitive understanding' of the analyst becomes all the more important. The RRM may be especially relevant for laconic participants.

Methods used to access reverie while examining transcripts

Just as writing a dream diary can stimulate a profusion of subsequent dreams, knowing the task is to track the reverie makes one more conscious of it. Although stimulated by the words on the page, at times the researcher seems barely aware of the transcript itself, focusing almost entirely on the developing reverie. There is a 'lost in the transcript' quality when this current is flowing.

Indeed, awareness of reverie while studying transcripts can be similar to remembering a dream – an image can leap into the mind, vividly, startlingly. Alternatively, an image may begin as a dim flicker that can be lost without sufficient awareness, or if the researcher is dismissive of his or her mental exploration in that moment.

The presentation of reverie in relation to interview scripts in 'final' written form may imply the sudden emergence of a fully-formed image, rather than a slowly evolving awareness. Also, when written down, reverie may imply a static image, but this is not always the case and where possible the more fluid feelings, fantasies and daydreams accompanying the experience need to be noticed and recorded.

It is possible that reverie will flow naturally into the researcher's mind while studying a transcript. But researchers can also feel stuck. It has been my experience, when teaching this method, that the following techniques can be helpful in stimulating reverie, should the researcher feel they are not forthcoming.

'*Squiggling*'. The psychoanalyst Winnicott's case notes are said to have consisted of small sketches he made at the end of sessions, an activity which probably has greater potential to retain or recreate symbolic exchanges in a psychoanalytic session than the written word (Kahr, 2017). Drawing a picture or making marks on the transcript before trying to find words to describe it, i.e. a 'squiggle game' (Winnicott, 1971) approach, can be helpful. (See Chapter 12 for an elaboration of the use of drawings in RRM.)

Identificatory internal role play. Imagining the researcher *was* the person speaking the words he/she has just read, including imagining what it felt in their body to have spoken the words.

'*Peripheral vision thinking*'. Being alert to what may have been unspoken, unexpressed and unspeakable.

Benign scepticism towards verbal responses. This assumes defensiveness as a normal response to the interview situation, and fosters a degree of scepticism of transcript words, especially when emotion is downplayed or avoided.

Acceptance of 'fuzziness'. If and when reverie develops, treating it as though a fish at the bottom of a clear lake. The key to keeping it in view is to tolerate cautious, manageable tension and uncertainty. We can't yet examine its scales, eyes, gills and tail, since getting too close will drive it away. And often the best that can be hoped for is a fleeting glimpse.

Creative elaborations. Imagistic responses to interview transcripts may often seem to be no more than an 'outline' of what the participant describes. For example, if a participant says she locks herself in her room and cries, we may picture just that. The 'reverie' entails paying attention to the creative adjustments we make – picturing her curled up in a ball, listening to music, sobbing into her hands etc.

Validation of the apparently irrelevant. Reverie may generate images which seem far removed from what is being said – in these cases it is important to allow the images to develop and not dismiss them.

Worked example of using RRM to analyse an interview transcript

Let's look at an example of how reverie can be used to facilitate novel understandings of research material. The interview here was with the mother of a depressed daughter. The reveries presented in the box at the top of this chapter and repeated below came to mind as she talked about her daughter's fears:

PARTICIPANT: She's absolutely (*said with emphasis*) terrified of me cos my mum died when I was 14, she thinks now when she hits 14, I'm gonna die and no matter how many times I tell her I'm healthy, I'm not going to die, she still thinks when she's 14 she – I'm not gonna be here …

INTERVIEWER: Hmm …

PARTICIPANT: So … I suppose there's a few things because from a young age, I always spoke about my mum, always – I took her up the hill like where she's buried for a couple of times so … and then she lost everything in the flood and then she lost *everything* (*said with emphasis*) again due to high levels of asbestos so everything she's ever owned has been taken away from her from a young age and then she built it all back up again and then it's all been taken away from her again …

> A sandcastle washed away by the sea. Clumps in the sand where it once stood. Soon, even these will be gone, wiped out by the waves, and flat sand will be left. '*I* [mother now speaking in the reverie] know what used to be there, but others may not'.

Where did this reverie come from? From the moment the participant said the word 'hill', I dimly pictured a bumpy formation. As the mother reiterates how things have been *repeatedly* lost, and the associated fear, the sea, with rhythmic predictability, entered the scene. Perhaps mother was saying that disaster inevitably, predictably, unavoidably, like the tides, dominates in her daughter's mind.

The sandcastle part of the reverie may be formed around the words 'built it all back'. Already I was imagining the sea, and to 'build a sandcastle' is a typical seaside thing to do. The reverie tells us that this sandcastle is in the process of dissolution: once a sandcastle, now it's a few lumps, and soon it will be flattened. This aspect of the reverie may be linked to the passing of life – the participant's mother's (the girl's grandmother's) death, the flood and the destruction it brought, physically and emotionally. Themes of burial and hiding link to this mother talking to her daughter about her own mother – what should and should not be said – the mother may be bearing some guilt for her daughter's suffering.

Using reverie to deepen understanding of research interviews

How does this reverie-informed analysis deepen our understanding of the interview? The researcher watches and listens to his/her reverie. The felt sense which the transcript excerpt evokes in the researcher is then linked back to the interview text.

In this case, the reverie was poignant, conjuring up childhood feelings of making sandcastles and – later in the day, with the tide rising – watching their destruction with a single powerful wave. In the interview text, the mother also talks about what is hidden beneath a bump in the earth – her mother's remains. Perhaps her daughter's 'absolutely terrified' state (from mother's point of view) is based on a tide-like predictability of death. Mother's reassurance ('no matter how many times I tell her I'm healthy') does not work ('she still thinks when she's 14 she's – I'm not gonna be here'). Perhaps all the daughter can hear is reassurance but her worry that the tide *will* come to wipe everyone out – now or very soon – remains.

The reverie of childhood playing in the sand now becomes a wait for impending horrors, just as perhaps the joyful, in-the-moment elements of the mother's own childhood were devastatingly interrupted. Another aspect might be the onset or impending onset of menarche in the daughter – the monthly 'tides', the possibility now of creating a 'bump' (i.e. pregnancy; also 'up the hill' could equal 'up the spout', a slang phrase for pregnancy), the mother's lack of having had a mother to guide her through her adolescence, and her worries about being able to do so for her daughter.

What is 'hidden under the earth' is a theme that emerges from this extract. Reverie generated a castle: an impregnable fortress – but in this case made of sand, and so liable to be swept away. Mum wants to hold onto her mother and keep her alive in both her and her daughter's mind. The reverie conjures up an attempt to deny the reality of loss. Perhaps now the daughter's depression can be seen as 'carrying' her mother's unresolved bereavement, and her justified fears about this will impact on her own development as a woman.

Research significance

A function of qualitative research is to generate hypotheses – often subtle, close-grained, experience-near ones. In the above example, there is an implicit hypothesis that adolescent depression needs to be seen in a familial and relational context, rather than being located in one 'ill' individual – the 'identified patient'. Fears about sexuality are integral to adolescent depression; maternal support is needed for the transition to sexual maturity to be accomplished. Without that support (possibly impeded by the mother's own adolescent bereavement), depression – in the sense of withdrawal and battening down emotional hatches – may be a 'safer' option than 'full catastrophe living' (cf. Kabat-Zinn, 2013).

More examples of RRM in data analysis

A possible criticism, to which I return in the next chapter, is that the RRM is a highly specialised approach, suitable only for the psychoanalytically initiated. In response to this I now show how the RRM can be used with interview transcripts which, at the data collection stage of live interviewing, were not in themselves RRM influenced. The interviews were not conducted by me; my only contact with the research data was through reading the transcripts. Equally, the interviewers had no knowledge of the RRM. These interviews were brief interviews undertaken with adolescents before they had had any therapy, but with the knowledge that they would be accessing this soon. Reverie is presented in box form, as above. Sometimes I drew a picture before attempting to convert it into writing (for example, in one case I drew a picture of a Petri dish).

Interspersed with interview text is some provisional and speculative understanding, which draws on reverie and links reverie experience back to the text. It is important to make clear that the thematic hypotheses generated here are presented in order to demonstrate the potential of the RRM. However, this is not to suggest that the presentations are sufficiently elaborated to reach authoritative research conclusions. Rather, this is a step in the data analysis process, and ideas for further work are explored in subsequent chapters.

Example 1: Tammy, aged 14: The father she dropped down the well

Tammy spoke vaguely about how she was referred to adolescent mental health services:

TAMMY: I dunno what happened like she [her mother] said er … I gotta start seeing a psychiatrist or sumfing.

INTERVIEWER: … do you think there's some things that you might be finding difficult at the moment?

TAMMY: Yeah, the only got of feeling difficult at the moment is just like my exams just gone, come round June, I'm gonna fail … cos I can't revise that easy …

I: Okay …

T: Like if I revise one night, I forget it by next morning, so now I always find it closer if I, erm, revise … in the morning or the next lesson or something …

I: Okay so you, it sounds like you're quite worried about your exams and you said that …

T: Yeah, my dad … my real dad he left – this year, September, it's gonna be 6 years since he left us …

> A stone falling down a well, Tammy's dad embodied, not being able to see down there, falling into nothing.

I: Okay …

T: And he – he hasn't sent us a new contact or … anyfink to let us know that he's okay.

We learn about Tammy's bleak outlook: 'I'm gonna fail'. She talks about her dad leaving; this followed her talking about her difficulty of holding onto information when revising. There is an out-of-control sense to both descriptions of her relationship to 'revision' and the physical absence of her father. Both may have felt 'there in the evening'. Her abrupt reference to her dad's disappearance may mirror what she felt about him leaving six years ago; it too was 'ab-rupt' (a rupture in her psyche), and not understandable, just as she does not understand how information she studies at night is erased by morning.

Were Tammy to enter psychotherapy, this 'here-today-gone-tomorrow' feeling about her dad may become a transferential theme. Tammy may be indirectly saying that therapeutic work will need to address the way she copes with these 'now you see it, now you don't' feelings. It could become important for the would-be therapist to make Tammy aware that he or she endures and survives in the days and nights between sessions.

Through reverie, new avenues of interpretation open up in response to the seemingly incongruous leap in the dialogue from exam worries to talking about her father. I thought about Tammy's possible feeling of being 'dropped' by her dad, but only after my RRM had pictured *him* as the embodiment of a stone falling into emptiness. There was a feeling associated with an image of 'he's there, somewhere, in the dark but it'll be a struggle to find him'. The image is ambiguous – is the well a bottomless pit, or is there a reachable foundation (as in the cover image of this volume)? Also, who dropped whom? The rapid change from her talking about revision to her dad primes us to the possibility that Tammy feels in some way responsible for him going out of her life. We do not have enough information at this stage to say this with authority, but the RRM provides the first step, capturing as it does both possibilities. Tammy gives an important sense of awareness of what is missing, and what should be there when she bemoans that her dad has not sent a contact address.

She continues to talk about her dad:

TAMMY: Yeah sometimes when I think that people erm people don't have much contact – contact with us, I feel like, like they've ended up in some type of accident or sumfing …

> The well becomes bottomless

T: … and we just don't know about coz he ain't bothered to call us or anyfing …

> The well develops a floor then the image transforms to dad lounging in a decrepit room, the phone next to him, him not thinking about Tammy

Reverie may make us wonder if Tammy is asking: 'does my dad love me? If he is dead maybe he did love me but I will never find his love – it has fallen off the edge of the earth.' This may even be preferable to the alternative, 'he's there, he's *choosing* not to contact me, in which case he may not love me at all'.

Tammy talks about her fears, which include dreams:

TAMMY: Yeah coz … if I do something nasty or like a scared dream, I have like flashback or like pictures in my head and it kind of puts me down in lessons when I have them …

When she says 'if I do something nasty or like a scared dream' it sounds as if she feels responsible for her dreams. I relate this to the dropped/dropper stone. Her words, 'puts me down', can be read as 'depressing me' and 'killing me' but also take us back to the well image, maybe in her mind she put her stone/dad down there. Perhaps, as mentioned above, Tammy is preoccupied with feeling responsible for her dad's departure.

I note that the Tammy at times picks up on the interviewer's words and uses them for herself, as though she is picking up the stones and throwing them in. For example, at one stage the interviewer mentions 'daydreams', and Tammy uses this word and expands on it. Although this could be taken as compliance, my feeling was that Tammy was picking up and adapting for herself the interviewer's words as though she was saying: 'you have found a way of saying/understanding things which I can use':

I: Okay, so is this when you're in Geography class and you're daydreaming and you get …

T: And then sometimes *I* just like daydream and it's that same thing and I have like a flashback or sometimes I close my eyes when it happens.

The interview continues:

I: … and what sort of things do you, do you do or what, how are you when you're feeling kind of vulnerable and kind of low?

T: not, I just feel like building up all tears inside me, and I feel bummed and feel like sitting in a quiet room watching a film to get my head away from it or something, not speaking to many people just sitting there computing …

> A well filling with water. Now the well becomes her throat and the water moves up her throat and mouth and silences her

Silenced by water/tears in reverie, this could be especially in relation to the feelings the conversation about her dad has aroused in her.

She goes on to describe her experience of being bullied at school. The way she recounts this as random cruelty took reverie back to the departure of her dad, and her dreams:

I: and what kind of things might you do when, when they've done that to you?

T: I normally just tell them that like wasting time, like it just … like my mum tells me not to listen to 'em but it's not my fault that I listen to 'em coz I try not to listen to them but they shout and everyfing, so …

> Her eyes are screwed tightly shut, her hands are over her ears, she's surrounded by a group of pupils in school uniforms violently leaning into her face, shouting at her. In her brain she hears the muffled, but clear shouts – she can't get away no matter how she tries

This 'not able to get away' began to emerge as a key to understanding Tammy's experience. Not only not being able to escape the bullies, she cannot get away from her depressed feelings, thoughts and daydreams. She cannot help listening to these bullies, just as she cannot help experiencing her frightening dreams.

What reverie added to understanding the Tammy transcript

The following emerged through using reverie responses to the script:

- Without reverie, Tammy's dialogue was hard to follow. Her words seemed incongruous and chaotic. Although Tammy seemed to struggle to 'logically' and verbally communicate, with the help of the RRM the interview transcript becomes rich with communication.

- Reverie provided links between forgetting her father and forgetting in her studies, and predicted forgetting the therapist between sessions. Reverie provided a vivid, concrete image – the dropped stone – suggestive of Tammy's feeling of having been 'dropped' by her dad.
- The image of the well led to the idea of her feeling trapped in her mind, of being controlled by her thoughts.
- Tammy's 'negative narrative' – what she was *not* seeing or understanding (revising in the night and forgetting in the morning, her father's absence) – came to consciousness. Data analysis strategies aiming to capture what is 'there' may have missed this 'present absence' – i.e. 'data' (revealed by reverie-aroused images in the researcher/transcript analyst) that 'hover' near the surface but cannot quite be put into words.
- The themes garnered through reverie led to the idea that a component of Tammy's depression is linked to feeling responsible – in part at least – for the departure of her dad.

This specific reverie data fits well with suggestions that when parents separate, the child may indeed feel in some way responsible (Wallerstein & Kelly, 1976), and that depression is often linked to an undue 'sense of control over good and bad outcomes' (Mirowsky & Ross, 1990, p. 71). The RRM provides qualitative evidential support for these clinical speculations, and generates further research questions which could be explored through RRM interviews with children in parent-absent families.

Example 2: Neil, aged 17: The powerful sun/son: life-giving, but also burning and desiccating

Neil had been a competitive figure skater before he suffered a serious injury. As I read the start of the interview, his words seem regimented ('I didn't feel happy at all and I didn't feel like I was any good at anything'), with little space for ambiguity, everything routinised like a skating drill. I note absence of reverie in myself as I read through the transcript. What little does arise seemed mere replication of his words:

NEIL: I went to the student counsellor because I wasn't really feeling too good with myself ... she referred me to the centre.

There is a sense of his wish to be independent and 'grown-up' which seemed to be achieved in his mind by not communicating his feelings. He mentioned 'throughout my life ... being really anxious' and 'having quite a lot of problems at home'. He said his stepmother and father argued a lot and his sister and father had 'verbal and physical fights'.

NEIL: They wouldn't know that, if I was depressed or anything, neither would any of my friends ... I wouldn't tell them.

There is some spark now perhaps, as Neil voices a psychological theory of his own impenetrability. This probably influences the first reverie experience below. Neil says that he is unwilling to speak of his depression but he is able to tell this to the interviewer. Asked by the interviewer why he would not tell his parents or friends if he were depressed:

NEIL: It doesn't help them [laughs]. I don't see … I don't think there's any need to tell someone something that doesn't benefit them.

> The sun – its rays giving growth

Paraphrasing, he says he cannot speak unless it is for the benefit of others. 'Not telling' would be enough to keep people out of his internal world. He does not believe that his family and those close to him will suspect something is wrong. Non-verbal communication is ruled out – if he doesn't tell them, they cannot know.

But reverie brought forth the sun. Neil may aspire to sun-like, life-giving existence. At this stage in the interview Neil is talking in quite a literal way. But this very barrenness reveals his internal object world, and may have been what stimulated researcher reverie to rush in and fill this affect vacuum.

The doubt that his certainty brings forth drives the reverie forward. As the interview progresses his position as the son/sun becomes more apparent. The interviewer asks him to expand, and his words and the reverie begin to develop:

INTERVIEWER: Ok, and where has that come from, your thinking?
NEIL: I don't know it just doesn't seem, doesn't seem right, like it doesn't … firstly I wouldn't tell anyone who's not close to me because I just don't think they'd care.

> A wilting plant – in the shade, beyond the sun's reach

Analysing the reverie, the initial sun imagery continues to illuminate the interview. We are finding out more about what kind of su(o)n he feels himself to be. The wilting plant links to the 'I don't think they'd care' phrase. It may be translated as: 'those whom I cannot touch, cannot care about me', emphasising a wish for self-sufficiency. But there is hope in his half-awareness that this is unrealistic: 'I just don't think …' He continues:

NEIL: I wouldn't tell anyone who's close to me because I don't want them to worry.

> Burning, leaves on fire

Now those close enough to be touched by him will be damaged. Suns scorch. If someone were to care about him and his unhappiness, in the reverie they are burnt by his worrisome needs. Like Icarus, they, or he, would be travelling too close to the sun/son. For others to worry about him would be destructive rather than helpful. The wilting plant is out of reach of the life-giving sunshine. This reverie came in the context of an emotion and sunshine-less family situation, with his warring parents and sister.

He continues:

NEIL: I don't want to look like er … I don't know that I can't handle myself or something.

> A plant growing on its own – a magic plant that doesn't need water – but it never actually grows, just stays stuck and static

I felt sadness for Neil, and the sorrowful isolation he conveys. Again there is hope in his hesitation and his words 'I don't want to look like'. Somewhere inside he doubts himself. In the reverie, the magic plant looks OK but never grows.

After noting this reverie, I was surprised to read what Neil went on to say: 'I feel that if I lived on my own that I'd be alright', as it seemed congruous with the reverie. Here is the complete extract:

NEIL: I feel that if I lived on my own that I'd be alright. But it's not everyday things like I can, I can work out how to wash my clothes and everything like that but um I'd erm … I don't really know what I want to do when it comes to getting a job and stuff like that.

> A dandelion with an infertile seed head

Theoretically the plant has the potential to reproduce, give life, but the reverie tells us that it is infertile, and will fail. This may be how he sees his adolescence: he can 'look after himself', but doubts whether he can grow into a man, or a father. The reverie seems largely focused on plants and their relationship with the sun. Plants are ephemeral, indicating a particular vulnerability apparent in Neil's dialogue. He may feel fragile as a flower, as he tries to assert himself, as a so(u)n.

Later in the interview Neil opens up more about his relationship with his father, and how he sees himself as different from him:

NEIL: Yeah, he talks about his emotions all the time, that's probably why I don't like to 'cos, I dunno, I just don't like to and he does.

A sunny Mediterranean courtyard. A water fountain – with a constant stream, and a dry pebble, near but not in the pool

I imagined Neil's dad as represented by this emotionally outpouring fountain, and Neil as the pebble. Neil feels held back and dry for not being able to let his emotions out and dislikes seeing his dad's emotional flow. The reverie image also contains a 'left out feeling' – the pebble on the edge of the pool. The earlier reveries of scorching sun and dry plants now take on new meaning – not only representing destructive forces, but also emotional desiccation. Earlier in the interview he had hinted that he would indeed like to be more emotionally expressive:

NEIL: I don't ever try to show my emotions to people.

One might expect someone to say 'I try not to'. But here we again have the sense that he worries about feeling overly in control of his emotions and that it would be an effort to show them. There is ambiguity. Neil may either be full of emotions and control them, or feel emotionally dead like the seed head of the dandelion (in botanical reality the 'dead' seed head is full of future life, but in my reverie it is 'infertile'). Is it an excess of emotion like his dad, or is he out of the sunshine, not growing, no more than a dusty pebble? Two bad options.

What reverie added to understanding

- Categories which might have been applied to the surface material such as 'privacy', 'desire for independence' and 'isolation' find symbolic expression through reverie – the *dry pebble*, the powerful and destructive *sun/son*.
- Neil's 'depression' (a conventional and contested term) is brought to life in the image of *fire* that either burns the people he touches or leaves cold those whom he does not, and in both instances denote isolation and lack of connectedness.
- The themes of *dryness and wetness* throughout the reverie can be understood as Neil's battle for emotional flow and richness, a battle which at this stage he does not want to engage in, but repeated hints suggest he does not feel comfortable in himself, for example in his language of pretence: 'I don't want to look like … I can't handle myself.' This ambiguity opens the space for reverie.
- His relationship with his father, which might have been noted as something like 'a fraught relationship' in non-RRM interview analysis, can be understood

in the context of Neil's battle for independence, his need to find his own *flowing fountain* (with its sexual overtones) within himself.

- A number of significant images arose through reverie in relation to Neil's situation: an unwatered plant; a sterile seed head; a dry pebble. Thinking about these – subjecting them to alpha function – the common theme is that of anxiety in relation to separation and subsequent generativity – 'Will I grow? Be able to share with another, marry, have children, be like my (over-)loquacious dad?'

Reverie aids our understanding of Neil's 'individuation' experience, a central challenge of adolescence, which can lead to depression if interrupted (Blos, 1967, 1968). This process seems to have been difficult for Neil. He talks about severing bonds with his parents brutally, abruptly, rather than growing naturally away from them. In Neil's mind, there may have been an absence of sufficient love. Rivalry and pain has predominated, especially in relation to his father. Reverie directs our attention to the notion that a parent has to 'be there to be left' (Furman, 1982, p. 15), and raises the hypothesis/core theme that adolescent depression may be a response to the challenge of 'leaving home' when developmental experiences and the relationship with parents have been problematic and in which overwhelming emotions have not found a 'home' where they can be contained and processed (Margaret Rustin, 2009).

Example 3: Sandy, aged 17: Alone in the Petri dish, watching the world dance

Sandy conveyed a sense of being out of control of her body:

SANDY: I couldn't go to sleep cos … I couldn't stop from shaking and I'd wake up in like these sweats.

She described an extremely troubled relationship with her father; she told the interviewer that her father would shout at her and tell her she was stupid and unattractive, and then Sandy said she felt 'sad … for letting him down'. She went on:

SANDY: Um I don't know … like my dad's health's been really bad mmm so he's kind of like … he had his … things in his ears as well … and it made his ears bad … and it made me feel more bad 'cos like I couldn't give him all the medication and then he blames it on me and said I did it on purpose.

Sandy as a slave to her tormenting father, chained to him

Earlier in the interview the reverie brought forth Sandy herself alone, sobbing, emaciated, desperate. Then the following interaction takes place:

INTERVIEWER: So you feel that you can't love him enough or you think he feels that?

SANDY: I know he feels it but I feel like I'm not enough …

A speck on a Petri dish

The reverie conveys a sense of being examined, and small, and of an existence in a sterile, lab-like condition, with nothing else and no escape. In the context of the problematic relationship with her father, this is a harrowing image. Another important theme emerges – that of feeling scrutinised by her father, who can still 'see' – Sandy feels – that she isn't good 'enough'.

She talks about the difficulties she has making friends at school. She says, 'I assume they're not gonna like me.' Then continuing the feeling that Sandy has an impoverished link with her father on which to build relationships, says 'so … that's why it's kind of hard to make connections'.

The Petri dish image morphs: a 'blob' on the dish: Sandy. Around her are other blobs that fuse and separate freely, they are dancing, alive. She remains a separate isolated blob

If Sandy is represented by this blob on the dish she is still a lonely and isolated figure. But she has grown from speck to blob. The reverie symbolised what it might feel like knowing that others *can* link and connect while she can't. By saying 'I assume that they're not gonna like me' she tells us that she has seen that people *can* link, like each other, play and connect. The image of her *chained* to her father takes on new meaning. There is a contrast between healthy fusion and separation compared to her experience of slavery and trappedness. After noting this image, I see that the next thing Sandy says in the interview is:

SANDY: I think it's how I'm feeling like even when I'm with people I still feel alone.

Later when she is asked if anyone knows about how she's feeling, she replies:

SANDY: Yeah family like they know it upsets me … but they're not, they don't really know.

Towards the end of the interview:

INTERVIEWER: … if you were to meet a therapist what would you kind of expect to happen? What would you like to happen?

SANDY: Um. I guess I'll talk to them, I would want them to help me stop thinking about things that make me sad really …

Shutters coming down, as in a bank robbery

At this point Sandy images that the best outcome would be for the sad feelings to be blocked from her consciousness. Shutters might link to her defence against the sad-making thoughts that penetrate her mind. In reverie, the therapist became the possible shutter mechanism. The mechanical element of this may be significant. A few lines later she herself uses the phrase:

SANDY: I want to be able to kind of shut people out. My dad.

The interviewer asks:

INTERVIEWER: to shut him out … to shut him out … what do you mean by to shut him out?
SANDY: Like so it won't affect the way I am

The blob on the Petri dish has become metallic; hardened, solid and impenetrable

This image opens up the fight between hardening, separating and accepting that her father is 'bad for her'. It is in contrast with the earlier, more hopeful image of needing to be able to soften and 'dance' with others.

What reverie added to understanding

- Reverie conveys a sense of chain-like 'bond' (with her father), but being able to see a glimpse of what a healthy relationship might involve, and what she might need to achieve that.
- The reverie suggests that there is hope (seeing the dancing other blobs) but the interview finishes on an ambiguous note with her feeling she knows what she needs – to break away from father – but seeming to think that this is only achievable by emotional hardening.
- Sandy seems to feel unbearably scrutinised. But she can 'see' that others don't seem to live in the misery which she inhabits. A feature of depression is that of invidious comparison and envy (Smith et al., 1994). Reverie shows Sandy's feeling of being 'under the microscope' and harshly judged.

The RRM here suggests a further hypothesis about adolescent depression – that external criticism is internalised in the form of depression, and how repeated negative appraisals can undermine self-esteem. Psychoanalytically minded therapists need to be aware of this as a possible element in transference, where 'interpretation' may well be experienced as criticism, thus reinforcing rather than alleviating depressive affect.

Discussion

I have attempted to show how the vivid image-based reverie responses to interview transcripts may result from feeling-contents 'housed' (Morgenroth, 2010, p. 277) in interview transcripts becoming accessible. Froggett & Hollway (2010) and Hollway & Froggett (2012) argue against social identity categories such as 'white, working-class', which close down the researcher's emotional receptivity to the unexpected. Hollway & Jefferson describe how their involvement in interview transcript analysis became more imaginative and emotional:

> working on the transcripts of a particular participant … we would feel inhabited by that person in the sense that *our imagination was full of him or her* … [and participants] *could appear in our dreams and waking fantasies.*
>
> *Hollway & Jefferson, 2000, p. 69, emphasis added*

The researcher's subjective experience is harnessed to further understand the ways in which standard diagnostic categories (e.g. 'depression', 'anxiety') play out as individuals' lived experience. The RRM approach to data analysis is made possible through 'affective and embodied experience' of the data (Redman, Bereswill & Morgenroth, 2010, p. 217).

Winnicott states:

> The precariousness of play belongs to the fact that it is always on the theoretical line between the subjective and that which is objectively perceived.
>
> *Winnicott (1968, p. 597)*

In these terms reverie can be characterised as a species of Winnicottian 'play'. The reverie approach goes beyond 'objective perception', but does not discount it. It is based on imaginative interplay between 'that which is objectively perceived' (i.e. the transcript text) and the subjectivity of the researcher's iterative reverie.

Conversations take place in chronological time, while feelings operate in an atemporal emotion-imbued rise and fall. Sequences in research interviews often seem illogical and irrational. If the researcher tries to bring order by ignoring, for example, the fact that Tammy jumped from topic to topic – from talking about revising to suddenly talking about her dad leaving – they may be left frustrated. By allowing reverie to pass through mind and body, the seemingly illogical may acquire meaning.

The technique offers the possibility of opening up and researching otherwise inaccessible aspects of participants' lived experience. In the Tammy transcript, the father embodied as a falling stone image suggested the possibility that Tammy felt responsible for his departure. When she says she 'does' a 'nasty or scared' dream, she verbalises this feeling of personal responsibility.

Through reading Sandy's account of her father's perception of her – 'I feel like I'm not enough' – we sense her pain. In RRM 'not enough' is represented as a 'scientifically' scrutinising judgement: she is an isolated blob on a Petri dish. With the help of reverie, Neil's depression and feeling of isolation arises out of his omnipotent, burning, sun-like self-definition. He fears his own power and doesn't want to burn the people he cares about with it, and so is condemned to isolation. RRM generates images that bring the sufferer's 'depression' alive, and stimulates further thinking and hypothesis-generation.

As research interviews can proceed in incomprehensible, illogical, non-linear ways, RRM can bring meaning to seemingly irrelevant phenomena. They are 'con-textualised' (i.e. 'textualised' together) in the intersubjective matrix. Decontextualised, reverie experiences might appear 'mad' and disconnected: what on earth have a Petri dish or the sun and wilting plants got to do with depression sufferers? Incorporating RRM into data analysis yields productive information about the texture and significance of experience.

In Sandy's interview, the RRM generated a personalised representation of experience. If incorporated into a treatment/outcome study, RRM qualitative data might encourage the therapist to help Sandy distance herself from her father without too much 'hardening', so that she could still be open to her friends' affection, while still caring about and for her father.

Reverie thus also may generate provisional theories surrounding potential transference relations. Tammy seemed to struggle with 'here today, gone tomorrow feelings' that could play out in therapy. RRM-influenced research might examine the clinical contention that countertransference and reverie experiences can predict aspects of an ensuing therapy (Margaret Rustin 2004), and therefore provide focal guidelines for therapists. In addition to its general applicability, it may be that the RRM is especially suited to studying aspects of psychotherapy and its outcomes.

The RRM emerged in the context of a study of adolescent depression. With the help of reverie, a number of core depressive themes emerged: feeling responsible for 'bad' things that happen (Tammy's dad leaving home); yearning for independence, but lacking sufficient base of love and support (Neil wants to separate but doubts his ability to 'be a man'); feeling intensely scrutinised and negatively judged (Sandy's preoccupation with being seen). In each case both a personalised picture of the participant's inner world and a tentative qualitative research 'finding' became accessible.

As discussed earlier, each reverie is unique: to the specific researcher and participant or transcript, and to the 'moment' of the reverie itself. The cases discussed represent just one researcher's perspective. Returning to Froggett & Hollway's (2010) account of scenic 'provocations', i.e. moments which 'register an emotional response', to increase a RRM-derived finding's validity it would be important to determine how this might vary for different researchers exposed to the same participant or transcript material. In the next chapter I explore this aspect by comparing a number of reverie responses in a group of researchers to the same extract from a research interview.

Conclusion

The method provides a means of drawing on and fostering the emotional links between researcher and researched. This method moves away from focusing exclusively on the verbal assertions of participants. The benefits, or 'value added', of this method are twofold. First, taking data analysis from *surface to depth*, and so potentially providing phenomenologically valid data about the lived experience of subjects. Second, *generating hypotheses* about the developmental and experiential origins of the phenomena under study (in this case adolescent depression) and thus pointing to further testable models and prevention strategies. In conclusion, adding a reverie dimension to transcript evaluation yields findings which have potential for incorporation into routine qualitative research methods, especially in the psychological domain.

11

RRM TEACHING GROUPS 1

General

The two previous chapters were based on my own reverie impressions and explorations. Crucial to the RRM is the idea that the value of reverie research is not confined to one person's musings but can be useful to the research community. But can reverie be taught? Some practices may enhance reverie, but does reverie, like 'mother love', have an innate quality? Since learning reverie is by its nature a personal journey, and since that journey must be at least in part an unexpected one, a traditionally didactic learning environment might be inhibitory. In this chapter I shall describe the evolution and practice of the RRM teaching group.

After attempting to systematise some elements of the reverie method for myself, the next step was to explore the applicability of the RRM for other researchers. An RRM teaching group was therefore set up which aimed to encourage reverie states of mind, and then apply it in research situations.

The teaching groups were made up of two contrasting sets of people. The first were young psychology graduates, working in various capacities on the same study of depression in adolescents from which the examples in the previous chapter were drawn. This group had little specialist knowledge of or interest in psychoanalysis. A contrasting group was made up of psychoanalytically oriented graduate students. As we shall see, this seemed to make a difference to how the groups responded to the RRM.

The groups provided an opportunity to study the wider applicability of the RRM. At the end of each teaching group, members were asked to independently study a section of a research interview transcript and employ reverie as they did so.

Thus the aims of these studies were to:

a) see if my own reverie-type experiences were generalisable to others;
b) study the impact of the training group, by observing whether reverie training enhances researcher sensitivity and so can provide extra depth and richness to interviewing more generally;

c) capture contrasts between the verbal manifestations of reverie in live research interviews and group discussion, and the private setting of studying a transcript, in which the researcher is 'listening to himself/herself'.

The RRM group aims to be a 'mutual experiential learning environment', in which people new to reverie researching can shape and compare their discoveries of reverie. A group approach also provides an opportunity to learn more about the processes and nature of reverie itself. I feel that the groups described below are a 'work in progress', and the reader may be stimulated in thinking about how to refine and improve them.

Psychoanalytic supervision: a brief digression

A significant strand in the thinking behind the reverie teaching group derives from the theory and practice of psychoanalytic supervision. Supervision of 'control cases' is generally regarded as an integral part of psychoanalytic practice (Kernberg, 2010). The supervisory relationship provides a forum in which the interpersonal events, conversations and countertransference are 'debriefed'. Supervision is typically a one-hour session, in individual or group format, in which the supervisee examines the minutiae of sessions with their patient, under the guidance of an experienced analyst/supervisor and colleagues.

The evolution of the theory of supervision parallels changes in the conceptualisation of countertransference described earlier. In the pre-Heimann phase, an essential component of supervision was to help analysts differentiate aspects of reactions and emotions deriving from their own unconscious from those of the patient. Analysts would be directed to bring those identified as 'belonging' to themselves to their training analyst, and/or to their internalised analytic process, or 'internal supervisor' (Casement, 1985).

The next phase, post-Heimann, was the recognition that the analyst's countertransference represents not just his/her unanalysed complexes, but, via projective identification, aspects of the patient's inner world, and that attending to these feelings in supervision provides an illuminating guide to understanding the patient. More recently, relational psychoanalysts have argued for supervision as a locus where, beyond the individual contributions of patient and analyst, their dialogic co-creation – the 'third' – can be brought into focus (Calgar, Bromberg & Meltzer, 2013). The supervisor–analyst relationship then becomes a 'second third', where the phenomena of the session – arising out of the inner worlds of patient and analyst – can be examined in the reflective space provided by the supervisor.

Ogden (2005a, p. 1265) has described the supervisory session as a type of 'guided dreaming', in which the supervisor provides a space in which the supervisee 'has time to waste' and is helped to 'fully dream' that which was blocked or inhibited in the possibly emotionally tumultuous environment of the analytic session. Ungar & de Ahumada (2001) similarly suggest that supervision provides a container for the emotional turbulence which contact with emotional disturbance arouses and enables it to be viewed with greater objectivity and differentiation.

Supervision and the RRM

The RRM groups aimed to offer a setting where researchers could consider their internal reactions as potentially relevant to the research encounter, in the presence of a group facilitator and other group members. Researchers working with the RRM without such a group may be at a disadvantage, but can nevertheless monitor reverie responses using their internal supervisory capacity, prior or current analytic experience and discussion with colleagues.

The justification for reverie researching rests on it being practically useful (e.g. in overcoming research blocks and obstacles or generating novel hypotheses), as well as theoretically beneficial. A wider question concerns whether reverie training has an effect on generic research interviewing technique, rather than in response to a specific participant or text, and whether it is helpful for qualitative researchers as a whole to be exposed to the RRM.

For reverie-enhanced research to be of systematic value, there should be parallels between different researchers' responses to similar participant-derived material. Given that no two RRM interviews can ever produce the same data, and will in many ways always be specific to that interview alone, this is an inherently problematic area for systematic, reproducible research. The standard solution is the 'inter-rater reliability' method, whereby two or more researchers study the same text, independently rate it and their responses are then correlated. The greater correspondence, the more reliable the data. Focusing on transcripts provides an analogue of this process for studying reverie. Group members – having experienced some reverie training – can be shown *the same* interview transcript, and asked to *independently respond, with reverie*. Comparing these responses lends support – or otherwise – for the validity and applicability of reverie data analysis, and evidence for reverie as a way of tapping into the intersubjective field.

Setting up RRM groups

A number of general principles inform the structure and format of RRM groups

Openness to the unexpected. In her classic book, *Drawing on the right side of the brain*, Betty Edwards (2008) suggests that good representational drawing is not possible if we have preconceptions about what it is we are drawing. She encourages a form of naive wonderment at the world – where, for example, the hand we try to reproduce is a collection of lines we have never seen before, and will never see again. From this perspective, we draw what we see slowly and carefully, and not what we think a 'hand' looks like, difficult though this is.

Thus too much 'explanation' may jeopardise the spontaneity that is the essence of the RRM. Participants are not offered too precise a definition of reverie, nor told in advance what the group will consist of. Group members are told that although some activities have been planned, there are no preconceptions about what their responses will be, and that each group is a unique event unto itself.

Silence and mindfulness. Participants are told that after each phase or demonstration, the facilitator will not necessarily talk in order to stimulate discussion, *nor* move on immediately, and that the groups are as much 'theirs' as 'his or hers'.

Meditation and mindfulness are now firmly in the mainstream psychotherapy agenda, with a proliferation of 'mindfulness-based' treatments (e.g. Grossman et al., 2004). A simple model of meditation involves sitting still, in a space without distractions, attempting to clear the mind of intrusive thoughts, and becoming aware of one's own breathing, or 'watching the breath'. This activity has demonstrable benefits, for example in inducing relaxation and reducing anxiety, and possibly reducing relapse rates in depression (Kuyken et al., 2008). As the RRM requires 'exploring in anxiety', meditative practice may well help the reverie researcher to realise that anxiety is transient and comes from within. Without wanting to simplify what is an immensely complex task, in theory, anxiety can then be examined as an object of interest, rather than being fled from (as one would from an external threat).

The psychoanalytic interest in mindfulness meditation derives from pioneers such as Erich Fromm's (1994) project of bringing together Western psychology with Eastern religious traditions. Meditation involves: 1) 'optimal awareness of the processes inside and outside oneself' (*ibid.*, p. 51) and 2) an 'insistence on independence and freedom' (*ibid.*). Fromm emphasises the link between self-awareness and empathy, i.e. 'other-awareness'. The aim is to move from the controlled, and largely solitary and largely non-interactional (at least at a verbal level), setting of meditation, to 'mindful living', described as follows:

> It means not to do anything in a distracted manner, but in full concentration of what is at and … it extends to every sphere of being: to the state of one's mind and to the mental contents of one's mind. Every experience, if it is done with mindfulness, is clear, distinct, real, and hence not automatic, mechanical, diffuse.
>
> *Fromm (1994 p. 51)*

The structural features required for successful meditation can be taken as precepts for a 'resting state' of inner stability. Their role is to act as the 'reins of reverie', somewhat analogous to the 'analytic setting' as the precondition for therapeutic work. Meditation is often initiated with the sound of a bell; here is my own description of this process:

> The chink of metal on metal. 'Waking' the bell – the second strike quickly climbs to a high-pitched, steady flow. Constant and mesmerising, like a spinning top: a black hole of sound. Now in slow descent, interweaving new sounds ring through. The sustain dances itself to silence, leaving an auditory afterimage – taken inside and into stillness. Awareness of the breath and heart beating in the chest. These automatic processes, usually unnoticed in normal waking life, fill consciousness, a reminder of in-the-moment being, and of the

> wonder, fragility and stability of being alive. Settling in, the breath becomes more regular. A tingling lightness passes through the body.

In teaching the RRM as an exercise to encourage calm and inner watching, group members are encouraged to sit still and 'watch the breath' for a few minutes, which provides the opportunity for heightened bodily awareness. The word 'meditation' is not usually used in the group training, however, as its spiritual connotations can be distracting. Rather, 'sitting still', 'quietly', and 'watching the breath' are phrases used to convey how 'not speaking' does not mean 'not doing', and that inner contemplation (symbolised by 'silence') can trigger creative receptivity.

Artistic receptivity. The arts may be conceived as 'shared dreams' (e.g. Gombrich, 1954, p. 402), where creator's and receiver's dream-worlds overlap. Some art may strike unconscious chords in the receiver where, like the mother's smooth-running alpha function, the stimulus is absorbed in a free way and is acknowledged and recognised but without needing to know explicitly what it 'means'. It may be useful in an RRM teaching group to provide a poem or image for the group to respond to.

Squiggle game. The aim at all times is to maintain the spirit of inner observation, but translate it into interpersonal communication. In the interview with Ann, reverie was viewed as a verbal analogue of Winnicott's 'squiggle game'. Based on this, the group members are invited to play the actual squiggle game in pairs, offering the chance to take part in a non-verbal 'conversation', where 'shared meaning is co-built' (Ferro, 2007, p. 1001) (Figure 11.1).

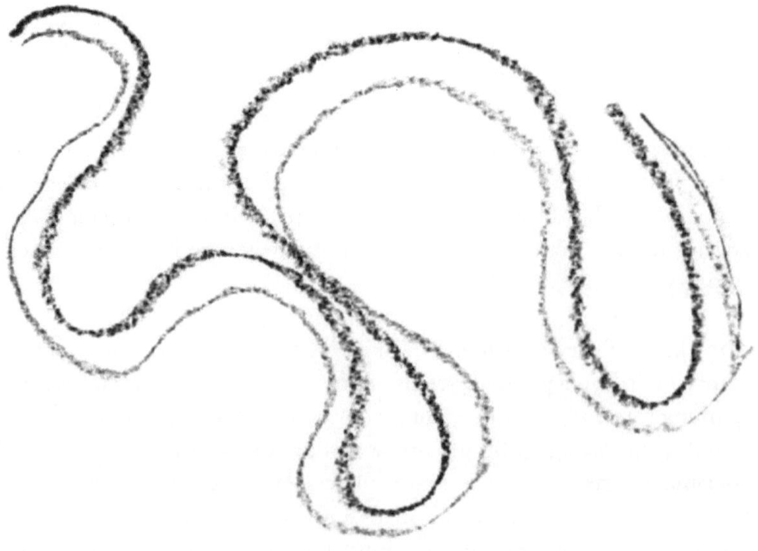

FIGURE 11.1 Squiggle A2: Group A squiggle.

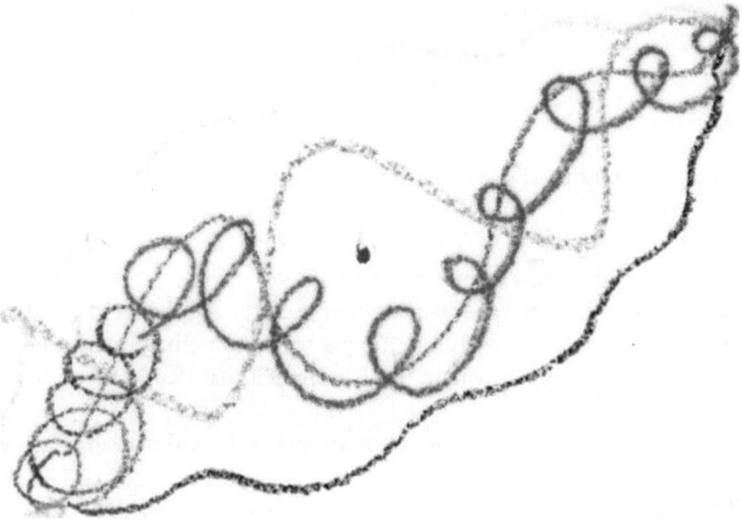

FIGURE 11.2 Squiggle A4: Group A squiggle.

For example, one 'squiggle' a pair worked on could be seen as representing an early-stage, trust-building reverie response based on mirroring, where one person's line has been made into a 'path' by the other – enabling them to 'walk together' (Figure 11.1).

This can be compared with another example from a different pair (Figure 11.2). There is an exploratory feel to this, reminiscent of the sea in its colouring, containing what may be seen as *controlled turbulence* – the central spirals to which both people have contributed (one in green, the other in dark blue). The relational culture seems to be of mutual support, where together the two participants can swim safely in the sea of anxiety which the uncertainty of the task evokes.

Specific phases of the groups

The aim is to create an ambiance for reverie, thereby setting the scene for reverie in relation to (although not limited to) research interviews. The early stages of the group require 'reverie priming' based on the exercises described above; a second section builds from this and looks specifically at the RRM.

Following these primers, the focus of the groups moves to research interviews. Participants interview each other in pairs (i.e. where a non-verbal squiggle could become verbal, about an unexpected topic such as 'the first birthday I remember'). Next, they individually complete a reverie-informed transcript analysis. The final element of the group consists of shared reflections.

As mentioned earlier, groups tend to respond differently depending on their level of psychoanalytic interest and sophistication. Here are some examples of such differences taken from tape-recorded sessions; Group B were the psychoanalytically more experienced.

Silences

Both groups brought up the issue of silence in the recorded reflections. One Group B member said:

FRANCESCO: … the silences are very good
SOMEONE: hmm (*in thoughtful sounding agreement*)
FRANCESCO: and, it I never felt like 'I need to say something, will it be alright if I – will it be ok if I just be silent?' Yes, I really felt that would be ok.

But for Group A, silence felt different – more pervasive and perhaps frightening:

ELLIE: … but um I have just felt – I don't like silences I don't like … I like to be told exactly what to do and what to say I don't like … (*now speaking more quietly*) doing things by myself, that makes me a bit uncomfortable …

Unsurprisingly, the psychoanalytically inexperienced Group A members found silence more threatening and inhibiting than their Group B counterparts.

Facilitator self-disclosure

In the service of creating an atmosphere of openness and 'story-sharing' (Heliker & Nguyen, 2010), as mentioned previously I have been influenced by the literature on 'social dreaming networks' (e.g. Eden, 2010), where people 'come together with the purpose of sharing their dreams and …. dream of issues and puzzles of common concern' (Lawrence, 2000, p. 85). In social dreaming, understanding may be reached when 'no amount of rational, cognitive exploration' could 'bring the same result' (*ibid*., p. 79). Eden describes the complexity of being both initiator and facilitator (i.e. in the scenarios below, me!), facing the competing tasks of managing the 'containing boundaries' of 'task, time and territory', while attempting to be 'alert to dreaming and free association' (2010, p. 181).

To demonstrate reverie in live interviewing, I asked the group to think of a scenario for me to talk briefly about. I had wanted this to be a spontaneous scenario so that I could not pre-plan my response. This modelled how an interviewee might feel in a research interview where they do not know what will come next. Group B asked me to talk about my first day at university. Here are my recollections:

> The group asked me to talk about my first day at university. My heart sank: imagining talking about my late adolescent self felt uncomfortably

revealing. I told the story more or less as follows, feeling rather a lot of internal chaos and noticing my anxiety, and worrying that it would fall flat:

> I was in the car with my parents. It was full of my 'things'. I sat in the back. I arrived at my halls of residence which seemed like an odd shaped house. The halls seem poorly located, close to a noisy recycling bin, and I felt annoyed at having followed my mother's advice about choosing which halls to live in. I met someone else who was to live in the halls. He looked strange to me, tall, 'Goth'-like, gangly, with an extreme Mohican haircut and a strong London accent. I felt like I'd been dealt bad luck and that I could never be friends with him (he ended up being one of my best friends at university!).

After some brief reflections from other group members there was silence. Feeling awkward, I was about to suggest we moved on, when Charlotte said quietly, with a hint of humour (perhaps because she thought it was so ridiculous) and embarrassment: 'well, I just pictured an old people's home'. I was struck by the feeling in Charlotte's voice and how this reflection had nearly slipped away. She said that she hadn't thought it was important. I admired her bravery in speaking. I asked if she could say more. She said:

> I went there [to the old people's home] when I was a child with a friend and we gave gifts to an old woman who I didn't know. It felt weird going there to visit this old woman who didn't even know who I was. She probably thought I was her granddaughter.

I suggested, perhaps over-enthusiastically hoping to convey that I valued her response, that this might link to my feeling about this unknown other, the person I didn't think there was a hope of being friends with. Charlotte nodded a little and fell silent.

Nevertheless, in the recorded reflections at the end of the group, Group B indicated that my participation helped them feel freer to join in, and talk about emotions:

LAINA: … I like the way you explored *your* memory … (*talking to me*) … I think that made us all feel a lot more comfortable

SEVERAL GROUP MEMBERS: Yeah!

FRANCESCO: Yeah that was really important yeah.

LAINA: And you were very accepting.

GROUP: (*lots of talking at once*) (*laughter*)

LAINA: We were shooting stuff out and, I was thinking – God he could – you could – he could get really offended with some of the stuff, like with, with for putting up with – like you did …

SOMEONE: hmm (*thoughtfully*)

LAINA: Like you took it really well
GROUP: hmm
LAINA: I think that made all of us feel really comfortable too
ISABEL: Ya, probably if you would've been very superficial about your memory we would've felt that's the way …

The conscious content of the above interchange seems to be the group expressing that the facilitator's self-disclosure helped them feel more comfortable to express their own feelings, and in the moment that this took place, it felt like a genuine expression of helpfulness. However, it is also possible that the above interchange indicates the difficulty in conducting such a group as one-off event. The somewhat idealised appraisal of the facilitator himself could have been in response to the apparently prevalent fantasy – not entirely misplaced – that the facilitator' self-disclosure involved 'putting up with' some inner conflict in relation to speaking about a personal experience. It is likely that the benefits of RRM teaching groups would be enhanced if there is the opportunity to have ongoing meetings throughout a research project, rather than a one-off.

Appraisal

Both groups seemed to find the process worthwhile, although there was greater hesitation and difficulty for Group A, especially in the early stages.

I did not formally ask for an appraisal, but such responses emerged naturally in the reflections:

I feel I've opened up a little bit more … I'm quite shocked at my own reaction … (Ellie, Group A)
I completely forgot … there was a schedule in the whole thing. (Kate, Group A)
I think it will make me look at transcripts in a slightly different way … develop the little things a bit more … I think this will kind of open it up. (Ellie, Group A).
I can't see – me bringing it into interviews. (Charlotte, Group A)
I didn't even feel tired which I normally do in lectures … [I felt] like free … to be and not to talk, or talk if I wanted. (Isabel, Group B)
I felt completely unforced, I think. (Rose, Group B)

RRM on RRM: fear of freedom

The RRM is intrinsically self-reflexive. It can be applied to several aspects of the research process: during the course of a research interview itself; when analysing transcripts; and at a 'supervisory' stage in responding to interviewers' reflections and comments. In the following section I use the RRM to think about the students as they reflect on the RRM group learning experience.

During the post-group recorded reflections, the groups were offered the chance to free associate around what they had experienced during the group. My own comments and reverie responses to their comments are recorded in the square brackets.

ELLIE: ... but um I have just felt – I don't like silences I don't like ... I like to be told exactly what to do and what to say I don't like ... (*now speaking more quietly*) doing things by myself, that makes me a bit uncomfortable ...

(*Sounds young, confidence stripped from her voice*)

[Ellie as a little child being led by the hand. I wonder if at this moment that she is in the midst of doing something by herself]

SOPHIE: I don't think I've given you what you want. Um and I'm just I suppose quite conscious of that really. Um, I don't think I could articulate exactly what you want. I don't feel like I've, I've done it.

(*Voice quietens as she says 'done it'*)

But ... I think that I would be aware – more aware ...

(*said as though correcting herself*)

... from now on in interviews when images do come into my head than I am ... I wouldn't always describe the moment the things that come into my head during interviews as images, they're just random thoughts, that I try 'n' suppress 'cos I'm supposed to be listening ... and it'll distract me but ... maybe actually the content of that thought isn't something to just suppress straight away.

(*Says from 'but ... maybe actually' more quietly as if in contemplation*)

Both Ellie and Sophie describe a form of being 'more aware'. But there is an ongoing tension, as with Ellie's dialogue, between the safety of the known and the excitement of the new. Sophie encapsulates what this would mean in research interviews, to try to 'suppress ... random thoughts ... 'cos I'm supposed to be listening ... but ... maybe actually the content of that thought isn't something to just suppress straight away'.

The reverie response to Sophie and Ellie's struggle leads to a consideration of the difference between dependence and freedom. At the time, dependence may be 'winning'. For Ellie this took the form of 'I like to be told what to do' – or held by the hand; and for Sophie – when she talks about 'I'm supposed to be listening'. These responses in my own reverie led to a picture a 'parental' figure in the scene, guiding, protecting, but also potentially controlling and stifling of imagination.

These extracts give the sense of how silence, reverie and potentially creative thinking inevitably also evoke anxieties. Such responses co-exist in a push-pull tension with more positive and exciting thoughts about the usefulness of reverie. There seems to be a moment of unstable equilibrium in which each set of thoughts immediately evokes the other, as the subject is swayed to and fro. Both positions have their allure – the calming safety of knowing where you are, and the excitement of exploration. The very idea of reverie, playfulness, of even momentary exploration, evokes a counter-reaction of conformity and the need to stick to protocols. This could be a microcosm of depression, its rigidity and trappedness, but also potential for growth if loss and low self-esteem can be transcended.

It is almost as if the stronger the impulse to reverie, the greater the resistance it evokes. Acceptance of reverie may for some research-minded participants entail a reorganisation of previously cherished ideas about what constitutes scientific psychological research. In the absence of a strong guiding hand, 'superego'-type thoughts about what is 'correct' might supervene to maintain the status quo. These could represent a constraining cage rather than a facilitating container.

These discussions lead to the idea that a state of openness to reverie entails a degree of anxiety and vulnerability. Too much anxiety makes reverie inaccessible; too little fails to stimulate reverie in the first place. Reverie may then emanate from tolerable anxiety. The starting point for this is a sense of what might be called 'homeliness' – a safe place, or secure base (Bowlby 1988) from which to venture out into the world of the unknown implicit in reverie, and to return to if things become too threatening. The task of the facilitator is to finesse this balance, requiring awareness of defences against anxiety, respecting and accepting them, but also looking for opportunities to help group members to go beyond them.

Different kinds of anxiety and psychic defences were present in groups that are or are not versed in psychoanalysis. In both, reverie seems to emerge out of uncertainty, of which silence is a prime promoter. In the psychoanalytically more experienced group, members were able to appreciate how silence was a necessary precursor to reverie, and so for them it was appraised as less oppressive.

'Silence' can represent the freedom whence unbounded creativity springs (Bion, 1965), but also can be experienced as trappedness (Meredith-Owen, 2007, p. 395). As mentioned earlier, 'silence' does not just refer to the 'not spoken'; it also delineates an internal space for reflection. Silence represents both an opportunity for aliveness, and a taste of the unknown. The aim of the meditation part of the groups is to foster 'listening to the silence' (Lawrence & Long, 2010, p. 227). Words and drawings never fully capture the actual experience – the thing in itself. Perhaps that lack/loss/'death' has to occur, and be momentarily mourned, before the experience can be communicated.

For instance, in the reflective space, one non-psychoanalytic member, Ellie, talks about silence and discovery in the same breath: 'I feel I've opened up a little bit more ... I've never liked poetry ... I don't like silences ... I like to be told exactly what to do and what to say.' This may demonstrate how death and birth are both contained in discovery – mourning the past uncreative self in the very act of creation. Silence, while perhaps a precondition for creativity, is also intensely threatening.

As exploration gathers pace, defences set in. Feeling intersubjectively connected can become unbearable and sometimes needs to be brought back to less threatening feeling states. An assumption of 'me-ness' (Lawrence, Bain & Gould, 1996) or an 'inviolable pristine self' (*ibid.*) has been described as a defence against the 'continual strain of being alive in the world of human beings' (Ogden, 1991, p. 388) or the 'unbearable embeddedness of being' (Stolorow & Atwood, 1994, p. 243). The idea of 'losing one's ego' is often responded to with the 'horror' and 'fantasies of danger' that Lawrence (2010, p. 4) suggests. Recorded feedback sessions typically start with a 'me'-type comment. These vocalisations come after a period of silence and uncertainty about what the warm-up activity was 'for'. Perhaps the moment before a first silence is broken is when people feel most psychically isolated and vulnerable, and the 'me' comment represents an attempt to reclaim the ego.

So, using the RRM is potentially disturbing as well as creative. Reverie researching, like social dreaming, 'is less comfortable … because it involves … risk and trust' (Oeser, 2010, p. 9). It involves 'the courage to go beyond the existing and institutionalized domains of knowledge', in particular 'daring to allow the unbidden' (*ibid.*).

A challenge of the RRM is that it appears to run counter to conventional academic standards, which evoke the desire for a return to existing knowledge and to feel safe in the familiar. This is especially the case when group members have a background in undergraduate psychology. As one Group A participant put it:

ELLIE: this isn't something you do on a day to day basis, it's not the way I naturally think about things, so it's not a natural process … and I think doing this has just made me very aware of it and I've never really thought about it before and so there's been that is it right, is it normal, is this the sort of thing that everyone else is picturing and …?

Ellie says how *thinking about* the unexpected things that come to mind in relation to research interviews is 'not a natural process'. She accepts that preconscious thoughts are 'there' but it is more normal to *leave* them there, to avoid 'thinking about thinking', rather than see them as potentially meaningful and useful 'data'. She links this with feeling exposed and comparing herself to others. It is uncomfortable, especially in a research context, to feel that that could be 'never one meaning, or interpretation' (Lawrence, 2000, p. 88).

A link between 'dichotomous talk' and creative interpersonal reverie played out in the groups. Dichotomies are often anxiety-stimulated. When threatened, there is a tendency to fall back on this-or-that notions, including, from an Oedipal perspective, mother-*or*-father rather than mother-*and*-father. The latter is the ultimate source of creativity (i.e. our being) but in the world of Oedipal anxiety, can feel obscure, threatening and uncertain ('I am alone; they are with each other; there may be a new baby that will oust me').

Dichotomous thinking is both a springboard for interpersonal reverie and creativity, but also an anxious response to the uncertain nature of reverie. Often in Group A, just as a movement towards reverie was made, there was a pull in the other direction:

ELLIE: I think it will make me look at transcripts in a slightly different way though … maybe just develop the little things a bit more … I think this will kind of open it up – but – I don't know that I'd include it in anything.

In this statement Ellie seems to correct her thought mid-sentence – her desire for exploration is shut down as she says the word 'but' – as though the thought came in '*but* ... this is not what research is supposed to be like'. Even though groups generally respond to and value reverie, there remains the challenge, a continuing stimulus to further work: even if the truth, inevitability and ubiquity of reverie is accepted, to what extent can it be played with and prove useful?

Conclusion

As with all new methodologies, if the RRM is to become part of more widespread interview technique a period of training will be needed. In this chapter I have described some of the group experiences that can help research groups begin to approach their interviews, both live and in transcript, in an RRM frame of mind. Now we move on to examining the effects of RRM groups on transcript analysis.

12

RRM TEACHING GROUPS 2

Data analysis

Having given a sense of the planning and atmosphere of the groups, let us now return to the specific research areas which the RRM groups explored: the impact of reverie research groups on using the RRM for data analysis.

Transcript analysis and RRM inter-rater reliability

In the earlier RRM work I was the only researcher involved. The intrinsic 'uniqueness' and specificity of reverie might suggest that replicability and generalisability – both somewhat complex in qualitative models – might be problematic if reverie is to be used more widely as a research tool. But given the theoretical basis of this research – that in intense dyadic encounters reverie may at times come into form as an *inter*personal phenomenon – there should be demonstrable links between one researcher's reverie response to a given script and another's. By exposing a number of different researchers to the same script and correlating their responses, RRM groups provide a forum where this issue can be explored.

More generally, the RRM teaching group provides a platform for exploring reverie transcript analysis. I'll now look specifically at two questions. First, can group members be encouraged to experience reverie responses to research material, and, if so, what is the nature of this reverie? Second, do these responses arise, in an 'intersubjective' manner, from the participant's material, and therefore have the potential to deepen, in a systematic way, understandings of participant interview responses, rather than merely represent individual researchers' idiosyncrasies?

I selected a two-page extract from an interview (the extract is presented at the end of this chapter, as Appendix 1). I had already studied this extract using the RRM, as described earlier. This enabled a further comparison to be made between group members' responses and my own. To recap, the transcript of Neil's interview brought up for me a reverie of the sun and its interaction with plants which seemed either to burn and make it wilt, or nourish it – but in my reverie, this 'nourishment' was felt to be 'inauthentic'. Themes potentially extracted without reverie might have focused on Neil's desire for self-sufficiency and independence, and his fraught relationship with his father. The reverie suggested a further understanding of Neil's internal struggle for emotional flow and richness. This reverie also suggested that for Neil intimacy may be connected to hurting, burning feelings, but that lack of intimacy is equally unpleasant, represented by dryness and distance.

I started by showing the group members a section of a different interview transcript (also described in Chapter 10) where I had drawn a dot on a Petri dish in the margin. I also showed them a question which had come to mind, which I had written beside this drawing: 'Does this capture a feeling of being examined, rather than free to be?' I showed them how, as the script had progressed, so the reverie had changed, when I had drawn several dots that were 'dancing' on the Petri dish.

Here I was attempting to demonstrate: a) how reverie responses *emerge* in response to interview transcripts; b) how these can be *represented* visually or verbally; c) how they can *change* as an interview progresses; d) how we can speculate as to the *meaning* of these reveries (i.e. to interpret) and attempt to link them to the verbal expressions of the interviewer and the interviewee.

I next introduced the participant in the transcript. I said it was an adolescent who had a diagnosis of depression (I did not mention the age or gender, hence why some of the reverie responses below indicate a female figure). I said the interviewer was not me, but another researcher. I then passed round a single sheet of paper. On it was the transcript excerpt. It was printed with wide margins and double-spaced, so providing space for participants to mark the page in whatever way they chose.

I explained that if images were experienced while studying the script, such images could be drawn, or described with words. I also asked them to mark on the script how they thought their responses might link with what is going on in the transcript (the attempt was to get the group members thinking about interpretative ideas relating to the transcript, which was described as 'reflections relating to understanding'). Speculation was encouraged, even if they judged their thoughts and reveries as irrelevant (cf. the 'fundamental rule', Freud, 1917c, p. 328).

Group members were asked to work independently on the transcript; 15–20 minutes were allocated for this process.

Data analysis. The transcripts annotated by group members were collected and studied. Data analysis took the following form:

1. Transcripts were studied individually, and initial impressions were noted.
2. Comparisons between transcripts were attempted. In the nine transcripts (five from Group B, four from Group A) certain sections of the script had seemed to stimulate more responses than others. I started noting similarities and differences between the scripts.
3. I brought in my own understanding of the transcripts and tried to see how this might link with, or depart from, what group members had written.

I was particularly interested in whether the reverie group could stimulate reverie in participants, what was its nature, and whether the reveries so generated indicate intersubjective communication, and therefore have the potential to deepen understandings of participant interview responses.

Is reverie experienced and what is its nature?

Responses range from reverie-absence, partial presence, to fuller reverie responses. *Near shut-down.* Some scripts are left almost unmarked, containing no more than a couple of words such as 'lost'. When this happens I sometimes feel a sense of responsibility, wondering whether further input is required for this participant in order to help reverie to flow.

'Replica' responses. To give an example, one respondee seemed to latch onto images from Harry Potter novels and films and kept 'seeing' them in ways that felt to me somewhat uncreative, but which (see below) were in fact consistent with the more spontaneous imagery that other group members produced. Also, this could be related to the sense conveyed in the transcript that the participant Neil may have at times struggled to feel authentically. It could be seen as a countertransference, or projective identificatory response, but without accompanying reflection.

Vague. Some scripts contained reverie such as 'a stuffed wallet', 'net', 'fledgling', 'a boy in his father's suit' reminding me of a 'patchy' dream. Here more work needs to be done to encourage speculations around the meaning of the specific reveries, and a greater understanding of the context and surrounding emotional atmosphere in which they have arisen. Without this reflective aspect, the reverie is intriguing but somewhat unproductive.

Dream-like. Some reveries are reminiscent of dreams. There is perhaps a 'two stage reverie' going on here – the group members' reveries and the facilitator (i.e. me) and his/her reveries to their reveries. This could be compared to an analyst's responses to an analysand's dreams, especially if they are working from an interpersonal position. For example, at one point in the transcript Neil says, 'I don't really know what I want to do next' and the following reverie was noted by a member from Group A:

> Looking lost – standing in a darkening playground, after everyone has left

The group member described what this meant: 'playground is (to me) the last place you walk when you leave school, so it's kind of that limbo of not being able to take the next step'. For me, the empty, darkening playground brought feelings of being the last child picked up from school, feeling different and less looked after. This in turn suggests that Neil's statement of not knowing what he wants to do next might also be a plea for help (an indication that he could benefit from therapy), as well as an expression of his sense of loneliness and the lack of a caring other.

Broaden and build. This describes reverie in which a series of images builds one on the another in a stepwise fashion. In this sequential pattern one image reinforces the previous, leading to a composite picture. For example, one participant wrote: 'Curled up on a single-seater sofa, knees drawn up (female)'. Then later:

> a more vividly isolated image, closing in on it almost:
> Dark around, on sofa, people in doorway – family/friends?

Here the reverie suggests a sense of isolation: 'single-seater', 'closing in', 'dark around', and painful separation from other people.

Discussion. In answer to whether reverie can be generated in response to interview transcripts, as suggested in Chapter 10, the answer is definitely 'yes'. Reverie-like responses are marked on most transcripts, and some group members are able to make tentative speculations about their meaning.

However, this exercise also clearly arouses anxiety and this sometimes leads to a shutting down – either completely, or immediately after a reverie had started to emerge. A distinction emerged between dreamlike reverie and more formulaic images which either stay rather close to the participant's words or become clichéd. Too much logic and order here seems to be a defence against the anxiety which unfettered reverie arouses.

Does the reverie indicate intersubjective communication?

A key question is in what way the RRM data analysis method affects the understanding of participants. For reverie to be a valid research method, it has to justify itself as an intersubjective process in which the participant's inner world interacts with that of the researcher. Are researchers' responses simply a manifestation of their own preoccupations, or do they tell us about the participant and their inner world and how it manifests itself intersubjectively?

Let's examine a small section of an interview and compare responses among group members. Two group members did not respond to this section. The other seven responses are presented below the text in boxes, whether verbal or drawn.

INTERVIEWER: So I don't know, what does that look like? So if I was to see you at home, you not feeling good, what would you be doing?

PARTICIPANT: I wouldn't be downstairs, I don't ever try to show my emotions to people … like I haven't told anyone, my parents know I come here, but they don't really know anything about me.

1.2A

Curled up on single-seater sofa, knees drawn up → Isolation, loneliness, in communal room but hidden by herself, feeling cut off

1.3A

Harry Potter in cupboard under the stairs

1.4A

'Everyone else is inside + she is alone outside – outside of the family home'

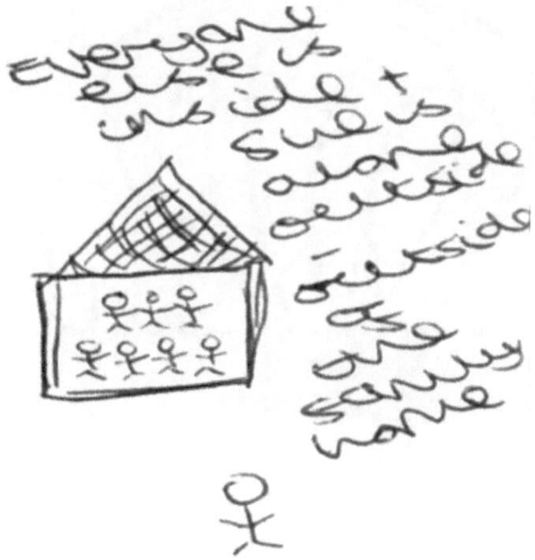

FIGURE 12.1

2.1A

Basement – dark, hiding

2.2A

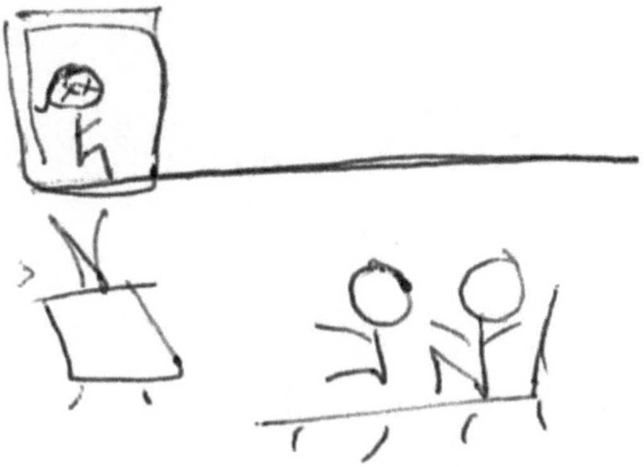

FIGURE 12.2

2.3B

Her alone in a corner of her room, on the floor, parents having fun downstairs

2.4A

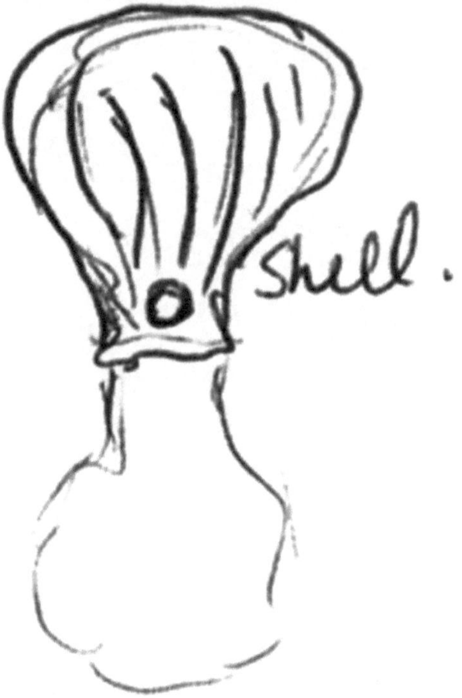

FIGURE 12.3

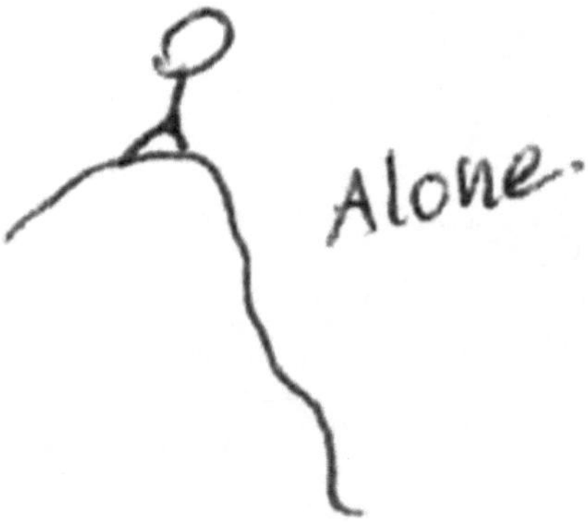

FIGURE 12.4

It seems indisputable that these responses were empathically evoked by the participant's words, and that they did not represent idiosyncratic responses belonging simply to the researcher and therefore scientifically irrelevant. In each reverie a sense of *a person, alone* is transmitted. The actual word 'alone' was used by three, and aloneness is implied in images such as being in a cupboard under the stairs, or on a 'single-seater' sofa. But given that a sense of feeling isolated is fairly explicit in Neil's words ('I don't ever try to show my emotions to people … I haven't told anyone') – does reverie add anything valuable?

I argue that representations of aloneness as accessed through the RRM provide avenues of *opportunity for understanding* this participant's feelings in greater depth. The reverie responses evoke multiple interpretations of aloneness. In the reveries, aloneness is concretely represented by specific images: out on a cliff face or outside the family home. The cliff is an open space, the family home a contained place – tantalisingly close yet still isolated. An alternative sense of aloneness seems to see the participant as 'marginalised': in a corner or basement. This conjures up a different feeling, perhaps linked to being trapped. One group member captures both aloneness and trappedness in her adjacent drawings of a shell and a cliff. For others, the level of emotional distance described seems to have converted Neil into an outcast – on the cliff or homeless. Through the RRM we move from a rather abstract word – aloneness – to a more psychologically meaningful contrast between two negative states: *claustrophobic trappedness* on the one hand, and *exposed isolation* on the other.

Aloneness for some seemed to find expression as 'Oedipal' exclusion in the sense of a subject excluded from a mutually engaged couple. Neil hints at this but does not speak it directly in referring to his parents who know he 'comes here' (i.e. to therapy) but 'don't really know anything about me'. The reverie integrates two elements, unspoken but hinted at by Neil: feeling alone, and a unified parental couple from which he feels excluded. One respondee draws a stick person, with dead eyes, away from a couple of figures next to each other watching television. For another participant, aloneness is presented in relation to parents 'having fun downstairs'. Another wrote 'outside alone' and drew a family together inside.

Thus the idea of Neil's exclusion sets off associations in the researchers. In reverie, he is depicted as having parents who don't think about him, leave him with his suffering and are unaware of the pain he suffers. Of course, none of this is necessarily 'factually' true, or only true some of the time, but suggests the *unspoken emotional truth* about how Neil may be feeling in this moment of the interview. By introducing a sense of feeling 'left out of a parental couple' – with its 'Oedipal' implications – the reverie method takes us several steps beyond Neil's transcribed words on the data analysis page.

Aloneness also finds alternative expression through the sense of darkness which is conveyed in some transcripts: 'basement – dark, hiding', 'Harry Potter in cupboard', or the shell drawing, where it would be dark inside (although not included in this section, almost every other part of this researcher's transcript referred to darkness). Darkness was also prominent in my own reverie analysis of Neil. What was it about Neil's words that gave several researchers this? Was his general flatness and hopelessness a 'dark' mood state which researchers were picking up on? The phrase 'in the dark' may be relevant to how he describes other people's knowledge – or, rather, lack of knowledge – of him: 'I haven't told anyone'.

His parents are described as more in the shade than total darkness; aware of the practicalities ('they know I come here') but more important emotional elements remain hidden: 'they don't really know anything about me'. Darkness may have featured so prominently in the group members' reveries in relation to Neil's already-has-his-mind-made-up language of certainty ('I wouldn't', 'I don't'). This was noted too in my analysis of his transcript, where I wrote that everything was 'neatly routinised, as in skating drills'. The dark/light black-and-white dichotomy leaves little space for shade and uncertainty in his life, and might be problematic in relation to his therapy, which, arguably is about introducing alternative possibilities into the fixity of depressive thought processes.

Reading just a few words of an interview script sets off myriad associations in RRM-primed researchers. When channelled and recorded, researcher associations can take the participant material in a number of directions, but with a distinctive common theme. This links via reverie to a feeling-imbued sense of a participant, which can then be modified, discarded or elaborated by the participant's subsequent expressions. These represent otherwise inaccessible qualitative data, valid in themselves, which can be used to generate further research questions. This process is shown in data analysis of the next section of interview:

PARTICIPANT: They wouldn't know that, if I was depressed or anything, neither would any of my friends, I wouldn't tell them.

1.2B

IMAGE: dark around, on sofa, people in doorway, family/friends? ANALYSIS: More explanation has led to a more vividly isolated image, closing in on it almost

2.1B

Dark black curtain [this is scribbled but still legible ...] cloak ... wrapped black curtain

2.3D

Headphones, away from anyone, s/he doesn't belong, not sharing or trying to include them

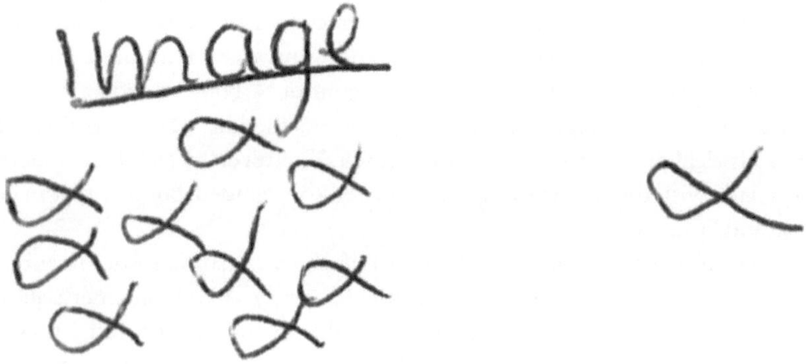

FIGURE 12.5

2.4C

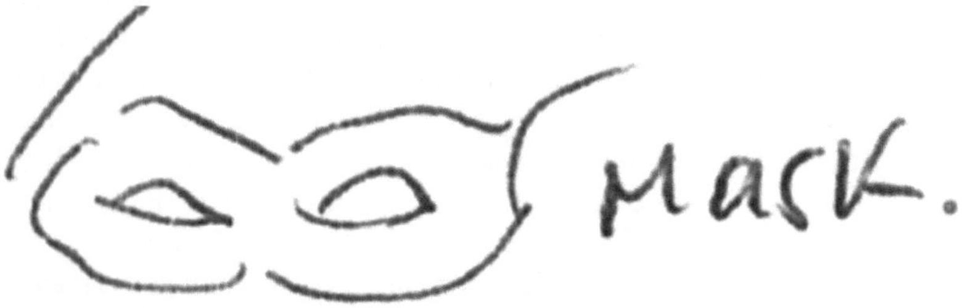

FIGURE 12.6

These reveries seem to shift the focus to a person *alone in relation to others*, as Neil explains how *no one can see* when he is depressed. For one group member, RRM brings up a fish swimming behind the others; another, whose original reverie was of the person on a single-seater sofa, now communicates a scene of an isolated individual surrounded by, but cut off from, friends and family. There is also a sense of hiding something or being hidden, *in the presence of others*: hidden in plain sight, either behind a mask, 'don't talk to me I'm wearing my headphones', under a cloak, behind a curtain or generally in darkness.

The cloaks, curtain, masks and headphones are tangible objects which have entered the scene in reverie (arising directly from group members' reveries, not Neil's words), which block him or hide him from human contact. They suggest an image of a child hiding, and of being an active agent in this hiding process – putting on a mask or headphones or covering himself in a cloak. This leads to the idea that Neil defends against his sense of helplessness by needing to be 'in control'. This links with my reverie of Neil's self-image as the sun that burns or gives life.

Through the accumulation of group members' reveries we can build up a symbolically expressed early impression of the participant's emotional experience. The feeling from Neil's first statement indicated irreconcilable aloneness, but the reveries suggest that with his second statement he wants the communication to shift towards relationships. Here his need to be in control – 'They wouldn't know ... if I was depressed ... I wouldn't tell them' – transmits the idea of unempathic others, and also his deliberate efforts to isolate himself. The reveries reveal an underlying *wish to connect* with the others from whom he felt so excluded, but fear that in doing so he would 'lose control'.

Let us return to the question of intersubjectivity versus 'autistic' reverie. The RRM includes a number of stages: creating a reverie-like 'container'; allowing reverie images, enteroceptive feelings and thoughts to emerge; recording these; and finally thinking about their meaning in relation to the participant and her/his difficulties. The evidence presented here suggests that there is indeed an intersubjective aspect to the group members' reveries, and that the RRM reveals useful additional data about participants, beyond the transcribed text. The researchers' responses did not merely reflect their inner worlds but linked meaningfully to the participant.

One can imagine that in a research project which was formally integrating RRM into its procedures there could be a similar process of reverie priming, followed by transcript analysis. Researchers could then reconvene and compare and contrast reverie experiences in order to build up a shared picture and understanding of an interview participant (cf. 'intervision', Marks & Monnich-Marks, 2003). This could then be incorporated into the data analysis and ultimately guide the way in which research papers are written.

In spite of the benefits of employing reverie-inspired methods at this stage of the research, there are also downsides. A concern might be that the creative elaborations around a participant take place at a relatively great distance between the researchers and the participant, and it is impossible to know what the participant him or herself would make of the interpretations. Thus while explorations may be freer and safer for this reason, they are also more remote.

To mitigate this, future studies might incorporate a form of 'action research' in which the research panel finds an analytic consensus in relation to an interview script, as mentioned above, but this time around which elements of understanding they wish to feedback to the participant, and this might inform a follow-up interview. Again, caution would need to be called for in deciding which elements, and how, to re-explore with participants and this would depend on the specifics of the research topic under consideration. The reverie method employed above creates a number of further possible research questions which Neil might be an interesting participant to interview in relation to, for example: 'adolescent males and their relationships with their fathers'; 'the drive for independence in adolescence'; 'feelings of Oedipal exclusion in adolescents' etc. In this way, the RRM in relation to preliminary interviews could be used as a sort of screen tool for suitability for a study; or alternatively, in retrospectively creating a research question.

Conclusion

This and the previous chapter suggest the following conclusions:

1. The reverie method can be taught.
2. Learning reverie can be threatening and evokes psychological defences to cope with the anxiety it arouses.
3. This anxiety at worst shuts down the reverie process, but, if manageable, stimulates it.
4. Reverie is meaningfully interpersonal in that a number of observers exposed to the same transcript material generate comparable imagery.
5. This imagery adds information about the affective state of participants.

Appendix 1

Extract from interview with 'Neil' which was presented to the group members:

I: So I don't know, what does that look like? So if I was to see you at home, you not feeling good, what would you be doing?

P: I wouldn't be downstairs, I don't ever try to show my emotions to people … like I haven't told anyone, my parents know I come here, but they don't really know anything about me.

I: Ok.

P: They wouldn't know that, if I was depressed or anything, neither would any of my friends … I wouldn't tell them.

I: Ok, and erm why is that, why wouldn't you tell them?

P: It doesn't help them (laughs). I don't see … I don't think there's any need to tell someone something that doesn't benefit them.

I: Ok, and where has that come from, your thinking?

P: I don't know it just doesn't seem, doesn't seem right, like it doesn't … firstly I would tell anyone who's not close to me because I just don't think they'd care and I wouldn't tell anyone who's close to me because I don't want them to worry but also I don't, I don't want to look like a er … I don't know that I can't handle myself or something.

I: Ok, and but do you feel that way, do you feel that you …?

P: No I feel that if I lived on my own that I'd be alright, but it's not everyday things like I can, I can work out how to wash my clothes and everything like that but I'd erm … I don't really know what want to do when it comes to getting a job and stuff like that, I don't know how, how I would …

I: Ok, so are these part of … like some of the things that have also been making you sad or …?

P: Yeah cos I don't really know what, I mean I'm near the end of year 13 and I don't really know what I want to do next.

I: Ok, so is that a concern for you?

P: Yeah.

I: Ok, and you mentioned you didn't want to let anyone know you were depressed, what do you mean by depressed?

P: Erm well the first time I came I did a questionnaire with (therapist) and he said only people that were depressed qualified and he said for the questions I … the way I filled out the questionnaire it qualified. So it was just the way I answered like my feeling of sad and not being worth and stuff like that … I sometimes wanted to hurt myself and stuff like that.

I: Ok, and do you feel that you are depressed.

P: Yeah, but it's not, it's not … I'm not all the time depressed, like it comes and goes, if I'm out with my friends and like having a really fun time I'd rarely ever would just start to think like depressive thoughts but pretty much every time I'm alone or at home or that I'll get that feeling.

13

DISCUSSION AND REPRISE

> Go some distance away because then the work appears smaller and more of it can be taken in at a glance, and a lack of harmony and proportion is more readily seen.
>
> *Leonardo da Vinci (cited in Kelly, 2004, p. 217)*

The moment has come to take a step back. The theme of this book and of the RRM generally is the balance between child-like 'free play of imagination' (Ferenczi, 1950 [1919], p. 189) and adult 'rational scrutiny' (*ibid.*). Researchers, as well as therapists, can draw inspiration from the triad: the *child* playing 'alone in the presence of *someone*' (Winnicott, 1958, p. 419), and the reflective *observer* (who may also be the 'someone'), thinking about both. Through 'being there' and 'letting be', while still 'managing the containing boundaries' (Eden, 2010 p. 181), the RRM allows research interviews to take their natural course. But, at some point, the researcher must step back and reflect on 'harmony and proportion', or their lack. There are parallels here with the practice and process of psychoanalytic supervision, in which the 'sturm und drang' of the session is recollected in tranquillity.

Here is another research prototype: a theme, etched into mind and body, lies dormant until reawakened in the living encounter of the research interview.

In an RRM group, Rose said:

> I really think that your own meaning is the only thing that stays with you anyway, 'cos like y'know after a couple years you're gun- … I will have forgotten everything, y'know the text books I've read and stuff … so I think that even like things like this group that y'know can look like mad on the paper maybe, is like the kind of thing that will be like – the actual crystal of knowledge that you … carry away, if it's something that you can translate into your own like … understanding.

Rose seems to be describing resonant researching where self-understanding develops in tandem with understanding the 'research questions' and the participants whose role it is to help answer them. This is a description of the quest for self-understanding as a springboard for interpersonal understanding. That, in essence, is the message of the RRM: aiming to help researchers to be 'objective about the subjective' (Hinshelwood, 2012, p. 136).

Reverie entered the psychoanalytic conceptual framework with Bion. His specialised formulation of reverie was an outgrowth of Freud's transference/countertransference model. But Bion (1962b) realised that transference and countertransference could both be seen as forms of 'waking dreaming'. Second, Bion saw that reverie was not necessarily narcissistic or other-excluding, but relational. Reverie is a vital component of mother/infant communication, and typifies the ways in which the mother, through her alpha function, transforms her infant's 'nameless dread' or 'beta elements' into thoughts which can be 'returned' to the infant, now detoxified and thinkable.

Moving from mother and baby to analyst and patient, Heimann (1950, 1960) realised that the analyst's countertransference was not so much an impediment but a vital indicator of the patient's inner world. To some extent, however, she failed to pick up on the mutuality implicit in Bion's model. For her, 'useful' countertransference was seen in terms of unidirectional projective identification. Bion's co-constructed bi-directional reverie is absent in her formulation. Winnicott by contrast was quintessentially a relationist. He theorised mother/infant mutuality in terms of healthy omnipotence on the part of the baby, and an attuned mother, primed through anticipatory timing to meet the baby's needs (e.g. Winnicott, 1971). Winnicott developed his own idiosyncratic theoretical framework of playful transitional phenomena and transitional space to account for this.

Amongst contemporary analysts, Ogden and Ferro have taken the field further. Both pick up on Bion's 'waking dreaming', but apply it to the analytic situation in somewhat different ways. For Ogden (e.g. 1997b, 1997c) the point of maximum therapeutic leverage in a session are the co-constructed waking-dreaming 'moments' of reverie which constitute an autonomous 'third', distinct from either party, available for thinking and transformation. For Ferro, the everyday conversation of the analytic session represents a 'narrative derivative' (Ferro, 2002) of the transference/countertransference matrix or 'field'; the task of the analyst is to use her/his intuition and clinical experience to penetrate to this ever-present, yet elusive, layer of experience and tap into the thematic material which lies beneath.

Lorenzer's (1983) 'scenic understanding', although less well known in the anglophone psychoanalytic world, also points to the omnipresence of unconscious forces which shape everyday life (including research interviews), and to their relationality. In his psychosocial model, the latter is reflected both in the unconscious preconceptions and defences which the participants bring to their interactions, but also in the ways in which prevailing social forces reinforce or discourage different elements in the interaction. In the research setting the prevailing socio-political dominance of the 'masculine' and instrumental chimes with emotional constriction in researchers and participants. At worst, the result can be affect-impoverished data, banal conclusions and non-replicability. The research interview becomes a *commodity exchange* in a utilitarian framework in which participants become little more than sources of information, plundered to fulfil research aims, and duly rewarded with financial incentives. All this misses the potential for psychological research interviews to generate an intimate engagement. 'When two personalities meet, an emotional storm is created' (Bion, 1979, p. 247). The RRM tries to meet the technical and theoretical challenges inherent in storm research!

The RRM brings a 'feminine' (in the sense of containment and receptivity) dynamic into the research arena which takes account of unconscious forces and feelings. The RRM can be used to extend interviewing techniques and provide an additional source of qualitative data. Drawing on the model of psychoanalytic supervision, especially in its less didactic form (cf. Basile & Ferro, 2008), this can be achieved even with psychoanalytically naive researchers.

In arguing for 'relational reverie', I have drawn on the idea of the 'third', developed not just by Ogden, but also Benjamin, Aron and other relationists. I have suggested that reverie as a state of receptivity is a psychic receptive space, arising out of both the patient's and the analyst's transferences, but with its own defining features. It represents a unique in-the-moment co-construction in which the analyst's empathic capacities are evoked by the patient's transferences to produce specific feelings and phantasies (typically imagistic).

There are of course dangers and caveats associated with the RRM. Freud was aware of the role and importance of the analyst's subjectivity – his countertransference – in empathically helping patients, but also of the dangers implicit in 'wild analysis'. In both analytic practice and the RRM, a range of feelings and fantasies will besiege therapists and researchers, outside of the control of the researcher, but usually full disclosure of this experience will be unhelpful. Some have argued that eruptions of raw affect need to be mediated and 'measured out consciously at all times' (Freud 1913, p. 112). But, experience may afford freedom: 'the surprise I experience in hearing my own voice is often a disconcerting one' (Ogden, 1998, p. 446). Ferenczi, Winnicott, Bion, Heimann all endorsed subjectivity in psychoanalytic technique. Like Freud, Winnicott was also cautious – ambivalent perhaps – about its misuse. He emphasises the privacy of the self:

> At the centre of each person is an incommunicado element, and this is sacred and most worthy of preservation.
>
> *Winnicott, (1965a, p. 187)*

Relational reverie

As well as Ferenczi, Bion and Ogden, another guiding spirit has been that of Erich Fromm, especially his ethical perspective on psychoanalysis, which I believe is also relevant to the research setting and to the subjectivity/objectivity tension. A thoroughgoing relational perspective cannot avoid the ethical – but also technical – question of the power differential between researcher and participant. A Foucaultian analysis of power differentials questions the possibility of researcher 'neutrality' (Cameron et al., 1993). 'Subject positions' (Edley, 2001) influence how researchers research and participants participate. Reflexive researchers are mindful of who they and participants are in relation to one another (Lucey, Melody & Walkerdine, 2003). Recent contributions raise the questions of 'who am I' and 'who are you' and extend sociological theorisations of researching (Froggett & Hollway, 2010). Hence the growing interest in psychoanalysis amongst qualitative researchers, as a discipline in which self-reflection is an indispensable tool for understanding intersubjective communication (Clarke & Hoggett, 2009).

While Freud may have publicly depicted psychoanalysis as a species of aseptic psychic surgery (Freud, 1917c), in private he was ready to acknowledge the necessary humanity of the analyst and interpersonal connectedness of the analytic relationship. His assertion that every analytic treatment was also a research enterprise (Freud 1912; Hinshelwood 2013) has to be seen in that light, and lends support to the qualitative, humanistic tenor which RRM strives for.

For a number of reasons, psychoanalytic reflexive paradigms have been viewed with caution by researchers. First, psychoanalysis has been marginalised within the scientific community (Stepansky, 2009). Second, the mutually incompatible-seeming array of psychoanalytic theories – Kleinian, Self-psychological, neo-Freudian, Independent – can be confusing, even to the initiated. Third, some psychoanalytic formulations might suggest that the analyst/analysand power differential, rather than being a hindrance or even a necessary compromise, is integral to the analytic process and even curative. From this perspective, the analyst's countertransference is the royal road to the truth, while the patient's phantasies emanate from neurosis and confusion. Could then there be a danger that psychoanalytically informed research legitimises researcher patriarchal dominance?

Perhaps the psychoanalytic concept most vulnerable to such a critique is that of 'projective identification' (Klein, 1946, p. 104), and its supposed 'unidirectional influence system' (Stolorow, Atwood & Orange, 2002, p. 88). One of the difficulties of cross-disciplinary studies is that contested concepts such as projective identification are adopted wholesale and the nuances inherent in *intra*-disciplinary debate can be missed. While in modern clinical practice many psychoanalysts adopt an approach compatible with the 'relational reverie' concept advocated here, using their evocative countertransference to track their patients' emotional states in the context of the in-session and in-the-moment relationship (Birkstead-Breen 2012), theoretical conceptualisations of the phenomena have lagged behind. The umbrella term 'projective identification' is often used to cover a number of distinct phenomena ranging from the expulsion of primitive mental states to the co-constructed 'third' which underlies the RRM.

From the RRM standpoint the 'third' can be seen as a) the co-constructed – 'healthy', playful – relational reverie of participant and researcher, unique to that conversation and distinct from the 'projections' and 'projective identifications' of either, and b) the reflexivity of the research enterprise itself where the aim is understanding not just the participant and her/his problems but also how the research procedures themselves contribute to the types of 'data' that are generated. RRM groups, comparable to psychoanalytic supervision groups, can help to build this reflexivity into research procedures.

Freud's public version of countertransference, with its connotations of precision and control, emerged at a time of psychoanalytic furore, in the midst of a battle between 'wild' analysis, represented by the extreme elements of Ferenczi's work, and the search for respectability and acceptance by a wider medical and scientific community, which was always Freud's hope. Later in the twentieth century, with growing interest in the earliest object relations, Klein and Bion drew on observations of mothers and babies. The theory of analytic reverie emerged in the context of reflections on mothering, play and creativity. Reverie comes alive not as a detached, reified 'analytic skill', but integral to 'what it means to be alive as a human being' (Ogden, 2001, p. 9).

Homeliness

Research happens at the boundary between the known and the unknown – the yet-to-be-discovered. Another theme latent in RRM has been that of the liminal. Creativity is produced at the 'frontier' (Ogden, 2001), 'won from the void' (Milton, cited in Bion, 1970, p. 151); a space both 'utterly empty, utterly a source' (Heaney, cited in Vendler, 2000, p. 112). Hence Ogden's doubly paradoxical, doubly liminal, definition of reverie: 'preconscious waking dreaming' (Ogden, 2004a, p. 1361) (i.e. neither conscious nor unconscious, neither waking nor dreaming).

Since reverie dwells in the liminal zone, it is only ever partially representable, with one foot in the tangible and describable, the other perpetually elusive. Psychic freedom – fresh, personalised responsiveness – is perhaps the central driver of creativity. When this psychic freedom breaks down, depression may ensue, a lifeless subservience. Creating out of freedom involves one's whole being, engendering a sense of potency and vibrancy. As we have seen, Freud, commenting this time not on dreams but creative writing, says that it 'arouse[s] in us emotions of which, perhaps, we had not even thought ourselves capable' (Freud, 1908, p. 173).

However, freedom is also 'healthily' retreated from, since in untrammelled freedom there is danger and a breakdown in the ability to distinguish dream and reality. Excessive freedom disrupts the sense of who one is, and what the world is. The will to freedom seems naturally balanced by an opposing pull towards safety.

However, defences may be instigated which 'punish' the push to freedom. RRM group members worried that using the reverie method might be somehow 'wrong'. From an Oedipal neo-Freudian perspective, the fantasised consequences of freedom contravene the patriarchal order; Lorenzer's model would suggest this anxious 'scenic understanding' reflected also the social taboo on freedom and feeling. Worries about scientific rigour, and students feeling that they should give the author, in his transferentially endowed position of authority, 'what I wanted', acted as a partial block on reverie. Here there is a similarity between the notion of 'parallel process' in the psychoanalytic supervision literature. This power relationship between researcher and participant can be played out in the reflexive group.

These benign defensive responses to freedom can be conceptualised in terms of the safety of the *intersubjective known*. This was earlier referred to as 'homeliness', in that it implies the importance of the familiar, comforting, predictable and recurrently returned to. Without the sense of somewhere safe to return to, dreaming and free association are potentially horrendous voyages. The RRM aims to establish just such a new home for psychoanalytically minded researchers.

Homeliness is an intersubjective, and vitally necessary, comfort rather than 'defence': away from isolation and Oedipal punishment, towards that which has, with luck, given us life and comforted us in terror. Poets, psychoanalysts and phenomenologists all and in different ways stress 'felt sense' (Perl, 2004), 'blood and bones' understanding (Lederach & Lederach, 2010), or corporeal intuition. This sense of being at home enough in one's own body to be aware of corporeal sensation, including discomfort, may be another precondition for reverie: 'I could feel in my body the patient's drinking in of every detail of the hallway' (Ogden, 1997b, p. 572). Primitive experiences of maternal holding are the developmental basis of homeliness.

In my interview with Ann – awash with flitting reverie; full of naive enthusiasm – I rush in to ask: 'do you know what your birth was like?' She looks shocked. I may not have been careful enough with the 'homely'. My question may have been a 'foreclosure of meaning' (Cooper, 1993, p. 95), prematurely directing the conversation. Questioning may have been experienced as a request for 'factual' details about her birth, and she obliged – and this may have reflected our need to return to familiar territory. As mentioned in that chapter, perhaps a non-interrogatory comment like 'when you said "birthmark", I imagined you as a baby being born' would have given Ann more of a chance to unconsciously work out how safe she felt before responding, or not. The originators of social dreaming stress the need for a 'homily' (homeliness's near relative, i.e. a reassuringly safe platitude) in getting their groups going, rather than silence or a pinning-down direct question: 'what is the first dream?' (Eden, 2010, p. 181).

For reverie researching to be useful and teachable it is necessary to embrace this paradox of the defence-freedom model. The unconscious is pre-verbal, preconscious, ineffable, yet the researcher is in search of 'findings'. Reverie is by its nature seen through a glass darkly. Qualitative researchers are well aware of this paradox: 'intuition without concept is blind: concept without intuition is empty' (Kant, cited in Coltart, 1986, p. 190). Within the growing tradition of psychoanalytically informed research, the RRM embodies a corpus of theory that attempts to respect both components of the 'intuition'/'concept' duality.

Reverie-informed qualitative researching

'Research interviewing' (Potter & Hepburn, 2005) entails a meeting between people, usually strangers, and attempting to facilitate and understand communications. Later the researcher finds ways of revisiting the encounter at the 'data analysis' stage, whether with the help of his 'internal supervisor' (Casement, 1985), or in a reflexive group setting. I have argued that researchers and participants may defend themselves from the emotionality of both the research interview and data analysis. Yet it is often precisely emotionality that is the object of qualitative research. The RRM aims to be an antidote to these dehumanising defensive tendencies (for further discussion see Michael Rustin, 2003, 2010), a step towards less defended, more reflexive researching.

It can be argued (perhaps rather late in the day for this volume!) that this striving is equally defensive. Perhaps my advocacy of the RRM is no less a defence against the anxieties associated with the fact that the human *subject* is also an *object*. Perhaps by focusing on the 'felt sense', dream and imagination, relationality, I am attempting to evade the brutal realities of the world. Against this, I have consistently argued that the emotionality of reverie is useful only if 'held' within an interpersonal field.

Qualitative research is constructed from 'languaged data' (Polkinghorne, 2005, p. 137). This neologism transmits the artificiality of language itself. But language is also an embodied manifestation of feelings. Words are entroceptively felt as they are said, formed by lungs, larynx, mouth, tongue and lips. This is the 'non-verbal' data source in qualitative researching. One aim of the RRM has been to move non-verbal data away from being talked about as supplementary, additional, a bonus, useful if noticed and to be noted where relevant. Instead, *the starting point for the RRM is the non-verbal.* For RRM researchers, reverie is not an optional 'add on', but is phenomenologically always in play. The issue is how it can be accessed, and how it can be used to foster research aims. If a research interview is viewed as a living interaction of two presences (Hyden, 2014), then every aspect of this interaction can become research 'data'.

Hollway & Jefferson, (2013, p. 151) have argued that psychoanalytically informed approaches to interviews can lead to an in-the-moment awareness of 'new thoughts'. But how are these 'new thoughts' to be instigated? I believe the framework of the RRM provides the necessary 'holding' for novelty to arise in ways that feel safe enough for it to be given voice. In research interviews, RRM researchers must strike a balance between supportive holding on the one hand and challenging the status quo on the other – their own and their participants. The RRM model – in live interviewing, data analysis and reflexive groups – aims to tread this subjective/objective tightrope.

Implications of reverie approaches for psychoanalytic researchers

Psychoanalysis likely must further embrace a research culture if it is to survive as a cultural and therapeutic presence (Stepansky 2009). Policy-makers and third-party funders want therapies which are 'proven' to 'work'. This seemingly legitimate requirement, arising as it does out of the 'drug metaphor' (Michael Rustin, 2003), misses the inherent complexity of psychological science. It runs against the position of 'healthy ambivalence' (Raphael-Leff, 2010), the possibility of multiple and personally defined truths, for example the integration of hate in loving relationships (Winnicott, 1949). Psychoanalysis finds itself in a bind – an evidence-base is essential to its survival (Fonagy, 2000), but narrow, utilitarian, instrumental versions of 'evidence' can run against its very essence.

Clinicians are concerned with the uniqueness of the individual, and the individual analysis. Case histories and psychoanalytic theorising typically do not meet conventional academic and scientific criteria for evidence, lack generalisability and tend only to be of interest to a fairly restricted group of like-minded practitioners. The RRM does not claim to solve the unsolvable but it has aimed to be a valid qualitative research methodology which places subjective and unconscious processes at its heart. My hope is that, with the help of the RRM, psychoanalytic skills can be brought to bear in a systematic way on research interviews and data analysis. I have tried to show how this can generate novel findings inaccessible to conventional research methods.

Of course, the RRM is no panacea. Reverie research, while of potential value to qualitative researchers wishing for alternative types of data and psychoanalysts in search of a discipline-congruent research method, has a number of limitations.

Most of the interviews described in this book were conducted with a specific population – adolescents who had experienced depression and either were about to receive, had received or were receiving psychotherapy. If the RRM is to establish itself more widely it will be important to explore the methodology with different populations, demographically and diagnostically, and across disciplines such as sociology and ethnography where qualitative research is the accepted paradigm. I hope the examples have shown how the RRM is useful not just in confronting verbal insufficiency, but that it can also help soften the defensive use of words in over-articulate subjects, bringing forth emotional themes that would be overlooked with a question-and-answer research format.

The roles of generalisability and replicability differ in qualitative research from its quantitative counterpart. The RRM fulfils the criterion of being a systematic, albeit complex, method of approaching both data collection and data analysis. Nevertheless, there is a wider question concerning the intrinsic individuality of the method. If every reverie is specific to a unique participant, interviewer and their interactions, how can we be sure that reverie-generated 'findings' are of general interest and applicability? The findings I have described in the preceding chapters go some way towards addressing this issue, in that different researchers exposed to the same transcript material generate comparable themes. This RRM 'limitation' is also a specific strength in that digging into the phenomenology of individual cases generates hypotheses of general interest which can be used to design future studies. In the case of Ann, a connection emerged between her history of birth trauma and depression. Whether this is a causal link or a 'narrative' one is debatable. The idea that a person's experience of depression is not just an 'illness episode' but is experienced by the subject as arising out of a specific life-history pattern needs to be tested in relation to further clinical samples.

Another unavoidable limitation of reverie researching is that it is time-consuming and therefore potentially costly in comparison with pen-and-paper research methods. The trade-off between depth and 'width' – i.e. numbers of participants studied – of a research method is difficult to finesse, but to the extent that reverie researching yields enriched data, the approach can be justified.

Methodology in qualitative research is a major area of debate and exploration. Many models and methods exist. The aim of this book has been to explore and expound the theoretical underpinning and practical guidance needed for using reverie in gathering and analysing qualitative data. Of course, this volume does not argue that *all* qualitative research should henceforth be reverie-based. But there is a case to be made that qualitative research, especially in the psychology field, could include at least one reverie-based interview. The data thereby generated will then raise impressions and questions leading to research hypotheses. I hope to also have shown how reverie-informed interviewing is a useful method for generating interesting conversations.

Epilogue

Reading Victor Hugo's *Les Miserables*, I come across a mini-study of reverie, of all things. The word leaps out at me in a chapter entitled 'The Field of the Lark' – as it had while reading Bion's two-page exposition in *Learning from Experience*. Perhaps reverie lends itself to such 'in-burstings' – which then fade, as does the meditator's bell, or the dream which falls away from our consciousness on waking.

If Bion, the polymath, read Victor Hugo – as he almost certainly did – he may have found inspiration for the psychoanalytic understanding of reverie from this passage:

> A certain amount of reverie is good … it soothes the fever … of the brain at work, and produces in the mind a soft and fresh vapour which corrects the too angular contours of pure thought, fills up the gaps and intervals here and there, binds them together and blunts the sharp corners of ideas.
>
> *Hugo (1950 [1862], p. 28)*

Although Hugo's description is 'intrapsychic' as opposed to RRM's interpersonal model, it describes a softened inner space, only a step away from homeliness as the springboard for the relational. As I read, my inner eye sees a raging infant, and mother approaching and embracing him. A 'soothing', cooling mist emanates from her being, as the child's distress subsides. Soothing and being soothed – 'affect co-regulation' – may lead to a fuller felt experience: 'the soul which loves and which suffers is in the sublime state' (*ibid.*, p. 29).

But Hugo also describes how, in excess, one can be lost to reverie, perhaps for evermore:

> Too much reverie submerges and drowns. Woe to the brain-worker who allows himself to fall entirely from thought into reverie! … Thought is the

> labour of intellect, reverie is its pleasure. To replace thought by reverie is to confound poison with nourishment … by continually going out for reverie, there comes a day when you go out to throw yourself in the water.
>
> ibid. *(p. 28)*

In Hugo's shocking warning against unchecked reverie – a potential route to suicide – I am reminded of Ann when she said: 'I like to piece myself apart' – a remarkably brave but frightening expression of fragmentation. Reverie can destabilise the psyche – putting us in touch with imperfection, dependence, helplessness and the near-unbearable realities of impermanence and death.

But to over-emphasise reverie's dangers is to do it a disservice. Reverie lies in wait, stalking the mind. By holding painful, fragmenting realities and bathing them in such 'soothing vapours', reverie can be coaxed into view; now we can begin to do some research. If we have a method, and I believe the RRM is one of them, for tolerating storms, we hear more clearly the sounds of the turning world, and our varied responses – painful, confused, avoidant, joyful – to them. And links begin to form.

REFERENCES

Adams, S. (1990). *The impressionists.* Philadelphia: Running Press.

Aguayo, J. (2011). 'Historicizing the paradigm shift in studies of countertransference: the world of Paula Heimann and Heinrich Racker', IPA Panel on British Object Relations and Countertransference, IPA Congress, Mexico City, 3–6 August 2011.

Aron, L. (1992). 'Interpretation as expression of the analyst's subjectivity', *Psychoanalytic Dialogues*, 2, 475–507.

Aron, L. (1995). 'The internalized primal scene', *Psychoanalytic Dialogues*, 5, 195–237.

Avdi, E. (2008). 'Analysing talk in the talking cure: conversation, discourse, and narrative analyses of psychoanalytic psychotherapy', *European Psychotherapy*, 8, 69–88.

Bajc, R. (2011). 'The power of art is the awakening of emotional communication', accessed online from www.sloveniatimes.com on 15 July 2012.

Balint, A. & Balint, M. (1939). 'On transference and counter-transference', *The International Journal of Psycho-Analysis*, 20, 223–230.

Barkham, M., Guthrie, E., Hardy, G. & Margison, F. (2017). *Psychodynamic-interpersonal therapy: a conversational model.* London: Sage.

Basile, R. (2006). 'Flaming Red: a session with Agnese', *International Journal of Psycho-Analysis*, 87, 629–635.

Basile, R. & Ferro, A. (2008). 'Some surprises: a new style for case discussion?' in: D. Tuckett et al. (eds.). *Psychoanalysis: comparable and incomparable.* London: Routledge, 234–242.

Basseches, M. (2005). 'The development of dialectical thinking as an approach to integration', *Integral review*, 1, 47–63.

Becker, E. (1997). *The denial of death.* New York: Free Press Paperbacks.

Beebe, B., Knoblauch, S., Rustin, J. & Sorter, D. (2005). *Forms of intersubjectivity in infant research and adult treatment.* New York: Other Press.

Bellow, S. (1975). *Humboldt's gift.* London: Penguin.

Benjamin, J. (1994). 'What angel would hear me? The erotics of transference', *Psychoanalytic Inquiry*, 14, 535–557.

Benjamin, J. (2004). 'Beyond doer and done to: an intersubjective view of thirdness', *Psychoanalytic Quarterly*, 73, 5–46.

Bereswill, M., Morgenroth, C. & Redman, P. (2010). 'Alfred Lorenzer and the depth-hermeneutic method', *Psychoanalysis, Culture & Society*, 15, 221–250.

Bergler, E. (1955). 'Contribution to the multiple meaning of psychogenic phenomena', *Psychoanalytic Review*, 42, 168–171.

Bick, E. (1964). 'Notes on infant observation in psycho-analytic training', *International Journal of Psycho-Analysis*, 45, 558–566.

Bion, W. (1959). 'Attacks on linking', *International Journal of Psycho-Analysis*, 40, 308–315.

Bion, W. (1962a). 'The psychoanalytic theory of thinking', *International Journal of Psychoanalysis*, 43, 306–310.

Bion, W. (1962b). *Learning from experience*. London: Karnac.

Bion, W. (1965). *Transformations: change from learning to growth*. London: Tavistock.

Bion, W. (1970). *Attention and interpretation*. London: Tavistock.

Bion, W. (1979). *Clinical seminars and four papers*. Abingdon: Fleetwood Press.

Birksted-Breen, D. (2012). 'Taking time: the tempo of psychoanalysis', *International Journal of Psycho-Analysis*, 93, 819–835.

Blass, R. (2013). 'Psychoanalytic controversy: introduction: what does the presentation of case material tell us about what actually happened in and analysis and how does it do this?', *International Journal of Psycho-Analysis*, 94, 1129–1134.

Blatt, S. (2008). *Polarities of experience: relatedness and self-definition in personality development, psychopathology and the therapeutic process*. Washington, DC: American Psychological Association.

Blos, P. (1967). 'The second individuation process of adolescence', *Psychoanalytic Study of the Child*, 22, 162–186.

Blos, P. (1968). 'Character formation in adolescence', *Psychoanalytic Study of the Child*, 23, 245–263.

Bogdan, R. & Biklen, S. (1982). *Qualitative research for education*. Boston: Allyn & Bacon.

Bollas, C. (1995). *Cracking up*. London: Routledge.

Bollas, C. (1998). 'Origins of the therapeutic alliance', *The Scandinavian Psychoanalytic Review*, 21, 24–36.

Bordo, S. (1987). *The flight to objectivity: essays on Cartesianism and culture*. Albany: State University of New York Press.

Bourdeau, B. (2000). 'Dual relationships in qualitative research', *The Qualitative Report* [Online serial], 4(3/4). Available from www.nova.edu/ssss/QR/QR4-3/bourdeau.html.

Bowlby, J. (1988). *A secure base*. London: Routledge.

Branney, P. (2008). 'Subjectivity, not personality: combining psychoanalysis and discourse analysis', *Social and Personality Psychology Compass*, 2, 2, 574–590.

Branney, P., Gough, B. & Madill, A. (2009). 'The other side of social psychology? A review of the utility of Lacanian psychoanalysis with a focus on the theory of the four discourses', *Annual Review of Critical Psychology*, 7, 187–204.

Braun, V. & Clarke, V. (2006). 'Using thematic analysis in psychology', *Qualitative Research in Psychology*, 3, 2, 77–101.

Brenman Pick, I. (1985). 'Working through in the countertransference', *International Journal of Psycho-Analysis*, 66, 157–166.

Briggs, C. (1986). *Learning how to ask: a sociolinguistic appraisal of the role of the interview in social science research*. Cambridge: Cambridge University Press.

Britten, N. (1995). 'Qualitative interviews in medical research', *British Medical Journal*, 311, 6999, 251–253.

Britton, R., Chused, J., Ellman, S. & Likierman, M. (2006). 'Panel II: the Oedipus Complex, the primal scene, and the superego', *Journal of Infant, Child and Adolescent Psychotherapy*, 5, 282–307.

Bunton, R. & Peterson, A. (1997). (eds.). *Foucault, health and medicine*. London: Routledge.
Burman, E. (1992). 'Identification and power in feminist therapy: a reflexive history of a discourse analysis', *Women's Studies International Forum*, 15, 4, 487–498.
Burnard, P. (1991). 'A method of analysing interview transcripts in qualitative research', *Nurse Education Today*, 11, 461–466.
Burnard, P. (1994). 'Searching for meaning: a method of analysing interview transcripts with a personal computer', *Nurse Education Today*, 14, 111–117.
Calgar, L., Bromberg, P. & Meltzer, J. (2013). *Clinical perspectives on the supervision of psychoanalysis and psychotherapy*. New York: Springer.
Cameron, D., Frazer, E., Harvey, P., Rampton, M. & Richardson, K. (1993). 'The relations between researcher and researched: ethics, advocacy and empowerment', in: D. Graddol, J. Maybin & B. Stierer (eds.). *Researching language and literacy in social context*. Bristol: Multilingual Matters, 18–26.
Canestri, J. & Fiorini, L. (2009). *The experience of time: psychoanalytic perspectives*. London: Karnac.
Cartwright, D. (2004). 'The psychoanalytic research interview: preliminary suggestions', *Journal of the American Psychoanalytic Association*, 52, 209–242.
Casement, P. (1985). *On learning from the patient*. London: Tavistock.
Casement, P. (2002). *Learning from our mistakes: beyond dogma in psychoanalysis and psychotherapy*. London: The Guilford Press.
Chessick, R. (1982). 'Metaphysics or autistic reverie', *Contemporary Psychoanalysis*, 18, 160–172.
Chiesa, M. (2010). 'Research and psychoanalysis: still time to bridge the great divide?', *Psychoanalytic Psychology*, 27, 99–114.
Civitarese, G. (2008). 'Caesura' as Bion's discourse on method', *International Journal of Psycho-Analysis*, 89, 1123–1143.
Civitarese, G. & Ferro, A. (2013). 'The meaning and use of metaphor in analytic field theory', *Psychoanalytic Inquiry*, 33, 190–209.
Clarke, S. (2002). 'Learning from experience, psycho-social research methods in the social sciences', *Qualitative Research*, 2, 173–195.
Clarke, S. & Hoggett, P. (2009). *Researching beneath the surface: psycho-social research methods in practice*. London: Karnac.
Clifford, J. & Marcus, G. (1986). *Writing culture: the poetics and politics of ethnography*. Berkley, CA: University of California Press.
Coffey, A. & Atkinson, P. (1996). *Making sense of qualitative data*. Thousand Oaks, CA: Sage.
Cole, E. (1922). 'A few "don't's" [sic] for beginners in the technique of psycho-analysis', *International Journal of Psycho-Analysis*, 3, 44.
Coltart, N. (1986). '"Slouching towards Bethlehem …" or thinking the unthinkable in psychoanalysis', in: G. Kohon (ed.). *The British School of Psychoanalysis*. London: Free Association Books, 185–199.
Cooper, S. (1993). 'Interpretive fallibility and the psychoanalytic dialogue', *Journal of the American Psychoanalytic Association*, 41, 9–126.
Crouch, M. & McKenzie, H. (2006). 'The logic of small samples in interview-based qualitative research', *Social Science Information*, 45, 4, 483–499.
Denzin, N. & Lincoln, Y. (2000). *A handbook of qualitative research*. Thousand Oaks, CA: Sage.
Denzin, N. & Lincoln, Y. (2011). *The Sage handbook of qualitative research*. Thousand Oaks, CA: Sage.
Deutsch, F. (1954). 'Analytic synesthesiology: analytic interpretation of intersensory perception', *International Journal of Psycho-Analysis*, 35, 293–301.
Devereux, G. (1967). *From anxiety to method in the behavioural sciences*. The Hague: Moulton & Co.
Dickson-Swift, V. (2007). 'Doing sensitive research: what challenges do qualitative researchers face?', *Qualitative Research*, 7, 3, 327–333.

Dooley, L. (1930). 'Psychoanalysis of the character and genius of Emily Brontë', *Psychoanalytic Review*, 17, 208–239.

Douglas, J. (1985). *Creative interviewing*. London: Sage.

Drisko, J. (2004). 'Case study research', in: D. Padgett (ed.). *The qualitative research experience*. Belmont, CA: Thomson Brooks/Cole, 100–114.

Eden, A. (2010). 'Learning to host a social dreaming matrix', in: G. Lawrence (ed.). *The creativity of social dreaming*. London: Karnac, 177–184.

Edley, N. (2001). 'Analysing masculinity: interpretative repertoires, ideological dilemmas and subject positions', in: M. Wetherell, S. Taylor & S. Yates (eds.). *Discourse as data: a guide for analysis*. Thousand Oaks, CA: Sage, 189–228.

Edwards, B. (2008). *Drawing on the right side of the brain*. London: HarperCollins.

Edwards, R. & Holland, J. (2013). *What is qualitative interviewing?* London: Bloomsbury Academic.

Ehrenberg, D. (1995). 'Self-disclosure: therapeutic tool or indulgence? Countertransference disclosure', *Contemporary Psychoanalysis*, 31, 213–228.

Eisenhardt, K. (1989). 'Building theories from case study research', *Academy of Management Review*, 14, 4, 532–550.

Ekman, P. & Friesen, W. (1968). 'Nonverbal behaviour in psychotherapy research', in: J. Shlien (ed.). *Research in psychotherapy*. Washington: American Psychological Association, 179–216.

Ellenberger, H. (1958). 'A clinical introduction to psychiatric phenomenology and existential analysis', in: R. May, E. Angel & H. Ellenberger (eds.). *Existence*. New York: Basic Books.

Elliott, H. (2011). 'Interviewing mothers: reflections on closeness and reflexivity in research encounters', *Studies in the Maternal*, 3, 1, online article.

Elliott, H., Ryan, J. & Hollway, W. (2011). 'Research encounters, reflexivity and supervision', *International Journal of Social Research Methodology*, online article.

Ellis, C. (2009). *Revision: autoethnographic reflections on life and work*. Walnut Creek, CA: Left Coast Press.

Ellis, C. & Bochner, A. (2000). 'Autoethnography, personal narrative, reflexivity: researcher as subject', in N. Denzin & Y. Lincoln (eds.). *The Handbook of Qualitative Research*. Thousand Oaks, CA: Sage, 733–768.

Ellis, H. (1919). 'The mechanisms of sexual deviation', *Psychoanalytic Review*, 6, 391–423.

Enckell, M. (1982). 'Film and psychoanalysis', *Scandinavian Psychoanalytic Review*, 5, 149–163.

Etchegoyen, H. (1991). *The fundamentals of psychoanalytic technique*. London: Karnac.

Etherington, K. (2004). *Becoming a reflexive researcher: using our selves in research*. London and Philadelphia: Jessica Kingsley Publishers.

Ezzy, D. (2010). 'Qualitative interviewing as embodied emotional performance', *Qualitative Inquiry*, 16, 3, 163–170.

Fairclough, N. (1996). *Language and power*. London: Longman.

Fenichel, O. (1939). 'Problems of psychoanalytic technique', *Psychoanalytic Quarterly*, 8, 164–185.

Ferenczi, S. (1910). Letter from Sándor Ferenczi to Sigmund Freud, September 28, 1910, *The Correspondence of Sigmund Freud and Sándor Ferenczi Volume 1, 1908–1914*, 214–215.

Ferenczi, S. (1932). *The clinical diary of Sándor Ferenczi*. Cambridge, MA: Harvard University Press.

Ferenczi, S. (1950 [1919]). 'Technical difficulties in the analysis of a case of hysteria', in: *Further contributions to the theory and technique of psycho-analysis*. London: The Hogarth Press, 189–197.

Ferenczi, S. (1955 [1928]). 'The elasticity of psycho-analytic technique', in: *Final contributions to the theory and technique of psycho-analysis*. London: The Hogarth Press, 87–101.

Ferro, A. (1993). 'The impasse within a theory of the analytic field: possible vertices of observation', *International Journal of Psycho-Analysis*, 74, 917–929.

Ferro, A. (2002). 'Some implications of Bion's thought: the waking dream and narrative derivatives', *International Journal of Psycho-Analysis*, 83, 597–607.

Ferro, A. (2007). 'Clinical implications of Bion's thought', *International Journal of Psycho-Analysis*, 87, 989–1003.

Ferro, A. (2009). 'Transformations in dreaming and characters in the psychoanalytic field', *International Journal of Psycho-Analysis*, 90, 209–230.

Ferro, A. (2011). *Avoiding emotions, living emotions*. London: Routledge.

Ferro, A. & Nicoli, L. (2017). *The new analyst's guide to the galaxy*. London: Karnac.

Finlay, L. (2002a). '"Outing" the researcher: the provenance, process and practice of reflexivity', *Qualitative Health Research*, 12, 4, 531–545.

Finlay, L. (2002b). 'Negotiating the swamp: the opportunity and challenge of reflexivity in research practice', *Qualitative Research*, 2, 2, 209–230.

Finlay, L. (2009). 'Debating phenomenological research methods', *Phenomenology & Practice*, 3, 1, 6–25.

Finlay, L. & Gough, B. (2003). *Reflexivity: a practical guide for researchers in health and social sciences*. London: Blackwell.

Flick, U. (2014). *An introduction to qualitative research*. London: Sage.

Flyvbjerg, B. (2006). 'Five misunderstandings about case-study research', *Qualitative Inquiry*, 12, 2, 219–245.

Fonagy, P. (2000). 'Grasping the nettle: or why psychoanalytic research is such an irritant', *The British Psycho-Analytical Society*, 36, 28–36.

Foucault, M. (1972). *The archaeology of knowledge and the discourse on language*. (A. M. Sharidan Smith, trans.). New York, NY: Pantheon Books.

Foucault, M. (1988). *Madness and civilization: a history of insanity in the age of reason*. New York: Vintage.

Franey, M. (2011). 'Book review: "… But at the same time and on another level …" Clinical applications in the Kleinian/Bionian mode (volume 2) by James S. Grotstein, M.D. London: Karnac, 2009; Volume 2, 286 pp', *Fort Da*, 17, 73–82.

Freud, A. (1937). *The ego and the mechanisms of defence*. London: Hogarth Press.

Freud, S. (1900). *The interpretation of dreams*. The Standard Edition of the Complete Psychological Works of Sigmund Freud (*S.E.*), vol. 4 (1900): *The Interpretation of Dreams (First Part)*, ix–627.

Freud, S. (1901). *The psychopathology of everyday life*, *S.E.*, vol. 6 (1901): *The psychopathology of everyday life*, vii–296.

Freud, S. (1905). 'Three essays on the theory of sexuality', *S.E.*, vol. 7 (1901–1905): *A case of hysteria, three essays on sexuality and other works*, 123–246.

Freud, S. (1908). 'Creative writers and day-dreaming', *S.E.*, vol. 9 (1906–1908): *Jensen's 'Gradiva' and other works*, 141–154.

Freud, S. (1909). Letter from Sigmund Freud to C. G. Jung, June 7, 1909. *The Freud/Jung letters: the correspondence between Sigmund Freud and C. G. Jung*, 230–232.

Freud, S. (1910a). Letter from Sigmund Freud to Sándor Ferenczi, October 6, 1910. *The correspondence of Sigmund Freud and Sándor Ferenczi*, vol. 1: *1908–1914*, 221–223.

Freud, S. (1910b). Letter from Sigmund Freud to C. G. Jung, February 2, 1910. *The Freud/Jung letters: the correspondence between Sigmund Freud and C. G. Jung*, 290–293.

Freud, S. (1910c). '"Wild" psycho-analysis', *S.E.*, vol. 11, 219–228.

Freud, S. (1911). Letters from Sigmund Freud to C. G. Jung, December 31, 1911. *The Freud/Jung letters: the correspondence Between Sigmund Freud and C. G. Jung*, 475–476.

Freud, S. (1912). 'Recommendations to physicians practising psycho-analysis'. *S.E.*, vol. 12, 109–120.

Freud, S. (1913). Letter from Freud to Ludwig Binswanger, February 20, 1913. *The Sigmund Freud–Ludwig Binswanger correspondence 1908–1938*, 112–113.

Freud, S. (1915). 'Observations on transference-love (further recommendations on the technique of psycho-analysis III)', *S.E.*, vol. 12, 157–171.

Freud, S. (1917a). Letter from Sigmund Freud to Karl Abraham, November 11, 1917. *The complete correspondence of Sigmund Freud and Karl Abraham 1907–1925*, 361–362.

Freud, S. (1917b). Letter from Sigmund Freud to Sándor Ferenczi, June 3, 1917. *The correspondence of Sigmund Freud and Sándor Ferenczi*, vol. 1: *1914–1919*, 211–212.

Freud, S. (1917c). 'Introductory lectures on psycho-analysis', *S.E.*, vol. 16, 241–463.

Freud, S. (1925). 'An autobiographical study', *S.E.*, vol. 20, 7–70.

Freud, S. (1931). Letter from Sigmund Freud to Sándor Ferenczi, December 13, 1931. *The correspondence of Sigmund Freud and Sándor Ferenczi*, vol. 1: *1920–1933*, 421–424.

Froggett, L. & Hollway, W. (2010). 'Psychosocial research analysis and scenic understanding', *Psychoanalysis, Culture & Society*, 15, 281–301.

Froggett, L. & Wengraf, T. (2004). 'Interpreting interviews in the light of research team dynamics: a study of Nila's biographic narrative', *International Journal of Critical Psychology*, 10, 94–122.

Fromm, E. (1994). *The art of being*. London: Bloomsbury.

Fromm, E. (2001). *Fear of freedom*. London: Routledge.

Frosh, S. & Baraitser, L. (2008). 'Psychoanalysis and psychosocial studies', *Psychoanalysis, Culture & Society*, 13, 346–365.

Frosh, S. & Emerson, P. (2005). 'Interpretation and over-interpretation: disputing the meaning of texts', *Qualitative Research*, 5, 307–324.

Furman, E. (1982). 'Mothers have to be there to be left', *Psychoanalytic Study of the Child*, 37, 15–28.

Gabbard, G. (1995). 'Countertransference: the emerging common ground', *International Journal of Psycho-Analysis*, 76, 475–485.

Gabbard, G. (2005). 'Joseph Sandler's contributions to the concept of countertransference', *Psychoanalytic Inquiry*, 25, 184–195.

Gadd, D. (2004). 'Making sense of interviewee–interviewer dynamics in narratives about violence in intimate relationships', *International Journal of Social Research Methodology*, 7, 5, 383–401.

Gall, J., Gall, M. & Borg, W. (2003). *Applying educational research: a practical guide*. New York: Longman.

Gemignani, M. (2011). 'Between researcher and researched: an introduction to countertransference in qualitative inquiry', *Qualitative Inquiry*, 17, 8, 701–708.

Gemignani, M. (2014). 'Memory, remembering, and oblivion in active narrative interviewing', *Qualitative Inquiry*, 20, 2, 127–13.

Georgaca, E. (2005). 'Lacanian psychoanalysis and the subject of social constructionist psychology: analysing subjectivity in talk', *International Journal of Critical Psychology*, 14, 74–94.

Gillham, B. (2005). *Research interviewing: the range of techniques: a practical guide*. Maidenhead: Open University Press.

Giorgi, A. (1970). 'Towards phenomenologically based research in psychology', *Journal of Phenomenological Psychology*, 1, 75–98.

Giorgi, A. (1985). *Phenomenology and psychological research*. Pittsburgh: Duquesne University Press.

Gitelson, M. (1952). 'The emotional position of the analyst in the psycho-analytic situation', *International Journal of Psycho-Analysis*, 33, 1–10.

Glaser, B. (1978). *Theoretical sensitivity: advances in the methodology of grounded theory*. Mill Valley: Sociology Press.

Gliserman, M. (1996). *Psychoanalysis, language, and the body of the text*. Gainseville: University of Florida.

Glover, N. (2009). *Psychoanalytic aesthetics: an introduction to the British School*. London: Karnac.

Goldman, R., Hunt, M., Allen, J., Hauser, S., Emmons, K., Maeda, M. & Sorensen, G. (2003). 'The life history interview method: applications to intervention development', *Health Education & Behavior*, 30, 5, 564–581.

Gombrich, E. (1954). 'Psycho-analysis and the history of art', *International Journal of Psycho-Analysis*, 35, 401–411.

Goodyer, I., Reynolds, S., Barrett, B., Byford, S., Dubicka, B., Hill, J., Holland, F., Kelvin, R., Midgley, N., Roberts, C. & Senior, R. (2017). 'Cognitive behavioural therapy and short-term psychoanalytical psychotherapy versus a brief psychosocial intervention in adolescents with unipolar major depressive disorder (IMPACT): a multicentre, pragmatic, observer-blind, randomised controlled superiority trial', *The Lancet Psychiatry*, 4, 2, 109–119.

Gough, B. (2004). 'Psychoanalysis as resource for understanding emotional ruptures in the text: the case of defensive masculinities', *British Journal of Social Psychology*, 43, 2, 245–267.

Green, A. (2012). *On private madness*. London: Karnac.

Green, D. & Latchford, G. (2012). 'Practice-based evidence', in: *Maximising the benefits of psychotherapy: a practice-based evidence approach*. New York: John Wiley & Sons, 87–108.

Grinberg, L. (1979). 'Countertransference and projective counteridentification', *Contemporary Psychoanalysis*, 15, 226–247.

Grossman, P., Niemann, L., Schmidt, S. & Walach, H. (2004). 'Mindfulness-based stress reduction and health benefits: a meta-analysis', *Journal of Psychosomatic Research*, 57, 1, 35–43.

Grotstein, J. (1979). 'Who is the dreamer who dreams the dream and who is the dreamer who understands it: a psychoanalytic inquiry into the ultimate nature of being', *Contemporary Psychoanalysis*, 15, 110–169.

Grotstein, J. (1984). 'A proposed revision of the psychoanalytic concept of primitive mental states, part II: the borderline syndrome, section 2: the phenomenology of the borderline syndrome', *Contemporary Psychoanalysis*, 20, 77–119.

Grotstein, J. (1995). 'A reassessment of the couch in psychoanalysis', *Psychoanalytic Inquiry*, 15, 396–405.

Grotstein, J. (2000). 'Reverie and interpretation: sensing something human', *Journal of the American Psychoanalytic Association*, 48, 628–631.

Gubrium, J. & Holstein, J. (2004). 'The active interview', in: D. Silverman (ed.). *Qualitative research*, second edition. London: Sage, 140–161.

Gubrium, J. & Holstein, J. (2011). 'Animating interview narratives', in D. Silverman (ed.). *Qualitative research,* third edition. London: Sage, 149–167.

Harris Williams, M. (2010). *Bion's dream: a reading of the autobiographies*. London: Karnac.

Heimann, P. (1950). 'On counter-transference', *International Journal of Psycho-Analysis*, 31, 81–84.

Heimann, P. (1960). 'Counter-transference', in: M. Tonnesmann (ed.). *About children and children-no-longer: Paula Heimann, collected papers 1942–80*. London and New York: Tavistock and Routledge.

Heimann, P. (1977). 'Further observations on the analyst's cognitive processes', *Journal of the American Psychoanalytic Association*, 2, 213–333.

Heliker, D. & Nguyen, H. (2010). 'Story sharing: enhancing nurse aide–resident relationships in long-term care', *Research in Gerontological Nursing*, 3, 4, 240–252.

Hess, N. (2000). 'Reverie and interpretation. By Thomas H Ogden. Karnac. Pp 295. £18.95', *Psychoanalytic Psychotherapy*, 14, 269–271.

Himes, M. (2001). 'Beyond the pleasure of the text: the writer and the reader', *Psychoanalysis and Contemporary Thought*, 24, 335–356.

Hinshelwood, R. (1997). *Therapy or coercion? Does psychoanalysis differ from brainwashing?* London: Karnac.

Hinshelwood, R. (2008). 'Melanie Klein and countertransference: a note on some archival material', *Psychoanalysis and History*, 10, 95–113.

Hinshelwood, R. (2010). 'Psychoanalytic research: is clinical material any use?', *Psychoanalytic Psychotherapy*, 24, 362–379.

Hinshelwood, R. (2012). 'On being objective about the subjective: clinical aspects of intersubjectivity in contemporary psychoanalysis', *International Forum of Psychoanalysis*, 21, 136–145.

Hinshelwood, R. (2013). *Research on the couch: single cases, subjectivity and psychoanalytic knowledge*. London: Routledge.

Holloway, I. (1995). 'Ethical issues in qualitative nursing research', *Nursing Ethics*, 2, 3, 223–232.

Hollway, W. (2009). 'Applying the "experience-near" principle to research: psychoanalytically informed methods', *Journal of Social Work Practice: Psychotherapeutic Approaches in Health, Welfare and the Community*, 23, 4, 461–474.

Hollway, W. (2011). 'In between reality and imagination', in: *Methodological Innovations Online*, special issue on multi-dimensional methods (eds. J. Mason & K. Davies). Accessed from www.esrc.ac.uk/my-esrc/grants/RES-063-27-0118/outputs/Read/f0ff90c5-f778-4127-bfcc-1434e1cd8b3f on 15 July 2015.

Hollway, W. (2012). 'Foreword', in: C. Urwin & J. Sternberg (eds.). *Infant observation and research: emotional processes in everyday lives*. London: Routledge.

Hollway, W. & Froggett, L. (2012). 'Researching in-between subjective experience and reality', *Forum: Qualitative Social Research*, 13, 3, accessed online from www.qualitative-research.net on 10 May 2018.

Hollway, W. & Jefferson, T. (2000). *Doing qualitative research differently: free association, narrative and the interview method*. London: Sage.

Hollway, W. & Jefferson, T. (2013). *Doing qualitative research differently: a psychosocial approach*. London: Sage.

Holmes, J. (2014). 'Countertransference before Heimann: an historical exploration', *Journal of the American Psychoanalytic Association*, 62, 4, 603–629.

Holmes, J. (2017). 'Reverie-informed research interviews', *International Journal of Psycho-Analysis*, 98, 3, 709–728.

Holstein, J. & Gubrium, J. (2011). 'Animating interview narratives', in: D. Silverman (ed.). *Qualitative research*, third edition. London: Sage, 149–167.

Hopkins, L. (2008). *False self: the life of Masud Khan*. London: Karnac.

Hugo, V. (1950 [1862]). *Les miserables*. Book Second. Trans. C. Wilbour. New York: Carleton.

Hunt, J. (1989). *Psychoanalytic aspects of fieldwork*. California: Sage.

Hurst, E. (1998). '*Psychoanalysis, Language, and the Body of the Text*. Martin Gliserman. Gainseville, FL: University Press of Florida, 1996. 196 pp.', *Modern Psychoanalysis*, 23, 119–124.

Hycner, R. (1985). 'Some guidelines for the phenomenological analysis of interview data', *Human Studies*, 8, 279–303.

Hyden, M. (2014). 'The teller-focused interview: interviewing as relational practice', *Qualitative Social Work*, published online first.

Jaspers, M. (1994). 'Issues in phenomenology for researchers of nursing', *Journal of Advanced Nursing*, 19, 309–314.

Jervis, S. (2009). 'The use of self as a research tool', in: S. Clarke and P. Hoggett (eds.). *Researching beneath the surface*. London: Karnac.

Jervis, S. (2011). *Relocation, gender and emotion: a psycho-social perspective on the experiences of military wives*. London: Karnac.

Kabat-Zinn, J. (2013). *Full catastrophe living: using the wisdom of your body and mind*, second edition. New York: Random House.

Kahr, B. (2017). *Tea with Winnicott*. London: Karnac.

Keen, E. (1975). *A primer in phenomenological psychology*. New York: Hold, Reinhart and Winston, Inc.

Kelly, M. (2004). *The rhythm of life*. New York: Fireside.

Kempf, E. (1919). 'The psychoanalytic treatment of dementia praecox: report of a case', *Psychoanalytic Review*, 6, 15–58.

Kernberg, O. (2010). 'Psychoanalytic supervision: the supervisor's tasks', *Psychoanalytic Quarterly*, 79, 603–627.

Kestemberg, E. & Zetzel, E. (1970). 'Discussion of 'Towards a basic psychoanalytic model'', *International Journal of Psycho-Analysis*, 51, 183–193.

Kincheloe, J. L. & McLaren, P. (2002). 'Rethinking critical theory and qualitative research', *Ethnography and schools: Qualitative approaches to the study of education*, 87–138.

Klein, M. (1946). 'Notes on some schizoid mechanisms', *International Journal of Psycho-Analysis*, 26, 99–110.

Kris, E. (1946). 'Freudianism and the literary mind', *Psychoanalytic Quarterly*, 15, 226–234.

Kuyken, W., Byford, S., Taylor, R., Watkins, E., Holden, E., Barrett, B., Byng, R., Evans, A., Mullan, E. & Teasdale, J. (2008). 'Mindfulness-based cognitive therapy to prevent relapse in recurrent depression', *Journal of Consulting and Clinical Psychology*, 76, 966–978.

Kvale, S. (1999). 'The psychoanalytic interview as qualitative research', *Qualitative Inquiry*, 5, 1, 87–113.

Kvale, S. & Brinkmann, S. (2008). *Interviews: learning the craft of qualitative research interviewing*. London: Sage.

Laplanche, J. & Pontalis, J. (1973). *The language of psycho-analysis*. London: The Hogarth Press and the Institute of Psycho-Analysis.

Lather, P. (2006). 'Paradigm proliferation as a good thing to think with: teaching research in education as wild profusion', *International Journal of Qualitative Studies in Education*, 19, 1, 35–57.

Lawrence, G. (2000). 'Social dreaming illuminating social change', *Organisational and Social Dynamics*, 1, 78–93.

Lawrence, G., Bain, A. & Gould, L. (1996). 'The fifth basic assumption', *Free Associations*, 6, 1, 28–55.

Lawrence, G. & Long, S. (2010). 'The creative frame of mind', in: G. Lawrence (ed.). *The creativity of social dreaming*. London: Karnac, 213–232.

Lederach, J. & Lederach, A. (2010). *When blood and bones cry out: journeys through the soundscape of healing and reconciliation*. New York: Oxford University Press.

Leider, R. (1983). 'Analytic neutrality – a historical review', *Psychoanalytic Inquiry*, 3, 665–674.

Leira, T. (1995). 'Silence and communication: nonverbal dialogue and therapeutic action', *Scandinavian Psychoanalytic Review*, 18, 41–65.

Lewis, I. (2008). 'With feeling: writing emotion into counselling and psychotherapy research', *Counselling and Psychotherapy Research*, 8, 1, 63–70.
Liamputtong, P. (2009). *Qualitative research methods*. Oxford: Oxford University Press.
Little, M. (1951). 'Counter-transference and the patient's response to it', *International Journal of Psycho-Analysis*, 32, 32–40.
Lorenzer, A. (1983). 'Sprache, Lebenspraxis und szenisches Verstehen in der psychoanalytischen Therapie', *Psyche – Zeitschrift für Psychoanalyse*, 37, 97–115.
Lorimer, F. (2010). 'Using emotion as a form of knowledge in a psychiatric fieldwork setting', in: J. Davies & D. Spencer (eds.). *Emotions in the field: the psychology and anthropology of fieldwork experience*. Stanford: Stanford University Press.
Low, B. (1935). 'The psychological compensations of the analyst', *International Journal of Psycho-Analysis*, 16, 1–8.
Lucey, H., Melody, J. & Walkerdine, V. (2003). 'Project 4:21 Transitions to womanhood: developing a psychosocial perspective in one longitudinal study', *International Journal of Social Research Methodology*, 6, 3, 279–284.
Marks, S. & Monnich-Marks, H. (2003). 'The analysis of counter-transference reactions as a means to discern latent interview-contents', *Forum: Qualitative Social Research*, 4, 2, accessed online from www.qualitative-research.net on 12 May 2018.
Mauthner, N. & Doucet, A. (2003). 'Reflexive accounts and accounts of reflexivity in qualitative data analysis', *Sociology*, 37, 3, 413–431.
Melles, G. (2005). 'Beyond the romantic impulse for authentic data to co construction of meaning in interview-based educational research', *Qualitative Research Journal*, 5, 21–30.
Meltzer, E. (2003). 'What's the matter with words? Vito Acconci's L-L-language of the written text', *Fort Da*, 9, 27–47.
Meredith-Owen, W. (2007). 'On evading analysis by becoming an analyst', *Journal of Analytical Psychology*, 52, 389–407.
Merleau-Ponty, M. (1962). *Phenomenology of perception*. Trans. C. Smith. London: Routledge & Kegan Paul Ltd.
Metman, P. (1957). 'The ego in schizophrenia, part II: Types and their treatment under consulting-room conditions', *Journal of Analytical Psychology*, 2, 51–71.
Midgley, N. (2003). 'Projective identification: a clinical exploration of the concept from a contemporary Freudian perspective', *British Journal of Psychotherapy*, 19, 4, 515–524.
Midgley, N. (2006a). 'Psychoanalysis and qualitative psychology: complementary or contradictory paradigms?', *Qualitative Research in Psychology*, 3, 3, 213–232.
Midgley, N. (2006b). 'The "inseparable bond between cure and research": clinical case study as a method of psychoanalytic inquiry', *Journal of Child Psychotherapy*, 32, 2, 122–147.
Midgley, N., Parkinson, S., Holmes, J., Stapley, E., Eatough, V. & Target, M. (2015). 'Beyond a diagnosis: the experience of depression among clinically-referred adolescents', *Journal of Adolescence*, 44, 269–279.
Midgley, N., Holmes, J., Parkinson, S., Stapley, E., Eatough, V. & Target, M. (2016). '"Just like talking to someone about like shit in your life and stuff, and they help you": hopes and expectations for therapy among depressed adolescents', *Psychotherapy Research*, 26, 1, 11–21.
Midgley, N., Parkinson, S., Holmes, J., Stapley, E., Eatough, V. & Target, M. (2017). '"Did I bring it on myself?" An exploratory study of the belief that adolescents referred to mental health services have about the cause of their depression', *European Child & Adolescent Psychiatry*, 26, 1, 25–34.
Milner, M. (1987). *The suppressed madness of sane men*. London: Tavistock Publications.
Mirowsky, J. & Ross, C. (1990). 'Control or defense? Depression and the sense of control over good and bad outcomes', *Journal of Health and Social Behavior*, 31, 71–86.

Mishler, E. (1991). *Research interviewing: context and narrative.* Cambridge, MA: Harvard University Press.

Mitchell, S. (1990). 'Discussion: a relational view', *Psychoanalytic Inquiry*, 10, 523–540.

Money-Kyrle, R. (1956). 'Normal counter-transference and some of its deviations', *International Journal of Psycho-Analysis*, 37, 360–366.

Montani, A. & Pietranera, G. (1946). 'First contributions to the psycho-analysis and aesthetics of motion-picture', *Psychoanalytic Review*, 33, 177–196.

Morgenroth, C. (2010). 'The research relationship, enactments and "counter-transference" analysis: on the significance of scenic understanding', *Psychoanalysis, Culture and Society*, 15, 3, 267–280.

Munhall, P. & Oiler, C. (1986). *Nursing research: a qualitative perspective.* Norwalk: Appleton-Century-Crofts.

Murphy, W. (1958). 'Character, trauma, and sensory perception', *International Journal of Psycho-Analysis*, 39, 555–568.

Noaks, L. & Wincup, E. (2004). *Criminological research: understanding qualitative methods.* London: Sage.

Oakley, A. (1981). *Subject women.* Oxford: Martin Robertson.

Oeser, F. (2010). 'Social dreaming to creativity', in: G. Lawrence (ed.). *The creativity of social dreaming.* London: Karnac, 9–23.

Ogden, T. (1991). 'Some theoretical comments on personal isolation', *Psychoanalytic Dialogues*, 1, 377–390.

Ogden, T. (1992). 'Comments on the transference and countertransference in the initial analytic meeting', *Psychoanalytic Inquiry*, 12, 225–247.

Ogden, T. (1994). 'The analytic third: working with intersubjective clinical facts', *International Journal of Psycho-Analysis*, 75, 3–19.

Ogden, T. (1995). 'Analysing forms of aliveness and deadness of the transference- counter-transference', *International Journal of Psycho-Analysis*, 76, 695–709.

Ogden, T. (1996). 'Reconsidering three aspects of psychoanalytic technique', *International Journal of Psycho-Analysis*, 77, 883–899.

Ogden, T. (1997a). 'Some thoughts on the use of language in psychoanalysis', *Psychoanalytic Dialogues*, 7, 1–21.

Ogden, T. (1997b). 'Reverie and interpretation', *Psychoanalytic Quarterly*, 66, 567–595.

Ogden, T. (1997c). 'Reverie and metaphor: some thoughts on how I work as a psychoanalyst', *International Journal of Psycho-Analysis*, 78, 719–732.

Ogden, T. (1997d). 'Listening three Frost poems', *Psychoanalytic Dialogues*, 7, 5, 619–639.

Ogden, T. (1998). 'A question of voice in poetry and psychoanalysis', *Psychoanalytic Quarterly*, 67, 3, 426–448.

Ogden, T. (1999). 'The music of what happens in poetry and psychoanalysis', *International Journal of Psycho-Analysis*, 80, 979–994.

Ogden, T. (2001). 'Conversations at the frontier of dreaming', *Fort Da*, 7B, 7–14.

Ogden, T. (2003). 'On not being able to dream', *International Journal of Psycho-Analysis*, 84, 17–30.

Ogden, T. (2004a). 'On holding and containing, being and dreaming', *International Journal of Psycho-Analysis*, 85, 1349–1364.

Ogden, T. (2004b). 'An introduction to the reading of Bion', *International Journal of Psycho-Analysis*, 85, 285–300.

Ogden, T. (2005a). 'On psychoanalytic supervision', *International Journal of Psycho-Analysis*, 86, 1265–1280.

Ogden, T. (2005b). 'On psychoanalytic writing', *International Journal of Psycho-Analysis*, 86, 15–29.

Olinick, S. (1982). 'Meaning beyond words: psychoanalytic perceptions of silence and communication, happiness, sexual love and death', *International Review of Psycho-Analysis*, 9, 461–472.

Osofsky, H. & Osofsky, M. (2009). 'Like father, like son: a psychoanalytical approach to interviewing in extreme circumstances', *Psychoanalytic Inquiry*, 29, 6, 529–541.

Oxford English Dictionary. (1997). Third edition. Oxford: Oxford University Press.

Paikin, H. (1995). 'From analytic dialogue to published text', *Scandinavian Psychoanalytic Review*, 18, 176–191.

Parker, I. (1998). *Social constructionism, discourse, and realism*. London: Sage.

Parker, I. (2005a). *Qualitative psychology: introducing radical research*. Buckingham: Open University Press.

Parker, I. (2005b). 'Lacanian discourse analysis in psychology: elements of theory and practice', *Theory & Psychology*, 15, 163–182.

Parker, I. (2010). 'The place of transference in psychosocial research', *Journal of Theoretical and Philosophical Psychology*, 30, 1, 17–31.

Parsons, M. (2007). 'An independent theory of clinical technique', *Psychoanalytic Dialogues* 19, 221–236.

Perl, S. (2004). *Felt sense: writing with the body*. Portsmouth: Heinemann.

Pile, S. (1991). 'Practising interpretative human geography', *Transactions of the Institute of British Geographers*, 16, 458–469.

Pistiner de Cortinas, L. (2011). 'Science and fiction in the psychoanalytical field', in: C. Mawson (ed.). *Bion today*. London: Routledge, 121–152.

Polkinghorne, D. (1995). 'Narrative configuration in qualitative analysis', *International Journal of Qualitative Studies in Education*, 8, 1, 5–23.

Polkinghorne, D. (2005). 'Language and meaning: data collection in qualitative research', *Journal of Counselling Psychology*, 2, 2, 137–145.

Potter, J. & Hepburn, A. (2005). 'Qualitative interviews in psychology: problems and possibilities', *Qualitative Research in Psychology*, 2, 281–307.

Rachman, A. (1993). 'Ferenczi and sexuality', in: L. Aron & A. Harris (eds.). *The legacy of Sándor Ferenczi*. Hillsdale, NJ: Analytic Press, 81–100.

Racker, H. (1953). 'A contribution to the problem of counter-transference', *International Journal of Psycho-Analysis*, 34, 313–324.

Raphael-Leff, J. (2010). 'Healthy maternal ambivalence', *Studies in the Maternal*, 2, 1, accessed online from www.mamsie.bbk.ac.uk/documents/raphael-leff.pdf on 15 March 2012.

Rapley, T. (2004). 'Interviews', in: C. Seale, D. Silverman & F. Gubrium (eds.). *Qualitative research practice*. London: Sage, 15–33.

Rapley, T. (2011). 'Some pragmatics of qualitative data analysis', in D. Silverman (ed.). *Qualitative research*, third edition. London: Sage, 273–290.

Redman, P., Bereswill, M. & Morgenroth, C. (2010). 'Special issue: Alfred Lorenzer and the depth-hermeneutic method', *Psychoanalysis, Culture and Society*, 15, 3, 213–214.

Reich, A. (1951). 'On counter-transference', *International Journal of Psycho-Analysis*, 32, 25–31.

Reik, T. (1933). 'New ways in psycho-analytic technique', *International Journal of Psycho-Analysis*, 14, 321–334.

Renik, O. (2004). 'Intersubjectivity in psychoanalysis', *International Journal of Psycho-Analysis*, 85, 1053–1056.

Riach, K. (2009). 'Exploring participant-centred reflexivity in the research interview', *Sociology*, 43, 2, 356–370.

Richards, H. & Schwartz, L. (2002). 'Ethics of qualitative research: are there special issues for health services research?', *Family Practice*, 19, 2, 135–139.

Richmond, V., McCroskey, S. & Hickson, M. (1991). *Nonverbal behavior in interpersonal relations.* Boston: Allyn & Bacon, Incorporated.

Ritchie, J. & Spencer, L. (2002). 'Qualitative data analysis for applied policy research', in: A. Bryman & R. Burgess (eds.). *Analysing qualitative data.* London: Routledge.

Rizq, R. (2008). 'The research couple: a psychoanalytic perspective on dilemmas in the qualitative research interview', *European Journal of Psychotherapy and Counselling*, 10, 1, 39–53.

Robben, A. (2012). 'The politics of truth and emotion among victims and perpetrators of violence', in: A. Robben & J. Sluka (eds.). *Ethnographic fieldwork: an anthropological reader*, second edition. West Sussex: John Wiley and Sons.

Roper, M. (2003). 'Analysing the analysed: transference and counter-transference in the oral history encounter', *Oral History*, 31, 2, 20–33.

Rosenblatt, P. (1995). 'Ethics of qualitative interviewing with grieving families', *Death Studies*, 19, 2, 139–155.

Rosenfeld, H. (1952). 'Notes on the psycho-analysis of the super-ego conflict of an acute schizophrenic patient', *International Journal of Psycho-Analysis*, 33, 111–131.

Rustin, Margaret. (1988). 'Encountering primitive anxieties: some aspects of infant observation as a preparation for clinical work with children and families', *Journal of Child Psychotherapy*, 14, 15–28.

Rustin, Margaret. (2004). *Assessment in child psychotherapy.* London: Karnac.

Rustin, Margaret. (2009). 'The psychology of depression in young adolescents: a psychoanalytic view of its origins, inner workings and implications', *Psychoanalytic Psychotherapy*, 23, 213–223.

Rustin, Michael. (2003). 'Research in the consulting room', *Journal of Child Psychotherapy*, 29, 137–145.

Rustin, Michael. (2010). 'Varieties of psychoanalytic research', *Psychoanalytic Psychotherapy*, 24, 380–397.

Safran, J. & Muran, C. (2000). *Negotiating the therapeutic alliance: a relational treatment guide.* New York: Guildford Press.

Sandelowski, M. (1995). 'Sample size in qualitative research', *Research in Nursing and Health*, 18, 2, 179–183.

Sandler, J. (1976). 'Countertransference and role-responsiveness', *International Review of Psycho-Analysis*, 3, 43–47.

Sandler, J. (1993). 'On communication from patient to analyst: not everything is projective identification', *International Journal of Psycho-Analysis*, 74, 1097–1107.

Sandler, J., Holder, A. & Dare, C. (1970). 'Basic psychoanalytic concepts, IV: Countertransference', *British Journal of Psychiatry*, 117, 83–88.

Schaeffer, N. (1991). 'Conversation with a purpose—or conversation? Interaction in the standardized interview', in: P. Biemer, R. Groves, L. Lyberg, N. Mathiowetz & S. Sudman (eds.). *Measurement errors in surveys.* New York: John Wiley & Sons, 365–391.

Scheurich, J. (1997). *Research method in the postmodern.* London: Falmer Press.

Schoenfeldt, M. C. & Schoenfeldt, M. (eds.). (2010). *A companion to Shakespeare's sonnets*, vol. 45. New York: John Wiley & Sons.

Seale, C. (2004). 'Replication/replicability in qualitative research', in: M. Lewis-Beck, A. Bryman & T. Futing Liao (eds.). *The Sage encyclopaedia of social science research methods.* London: Sage.

Segal, H. (1975). 'A psychoanalytic approach to the treatment of schizophrenia', in: M. Lader (ed.). *Studies of schizophrenia.* Ashford: Headley; reprinted (1981) as 'A psychoanalytic approach ot the treatment of psychoses', in *The Work of Hanna Segal*, New York and London: Jason Aronson, 131–136.

Segal, H. (1977). 'Countertransference', *International Journal of Psychoanalytic Psychotherapy*, 6, 31–37.
Seitz, P. (1966). 'The consensus problem in psychoanalytic research', in: L. Gottschalk & L. Auerbach (eds.). *Methods of research in psychotherapy*. New York: Guildford Press, 209–225.
Shakow, D. (1960). 'The recorded psychoanalytic interview as an objective approach to research in psychoanalysis', *Psychoanalytic Quarterly*, 29, 82–97.
Shamai, M. (2003). 'Therapeutic effects of qualitative research: reconstructing the experience of treatment as a by-product of qualitative evaluation', *Social Service Review*, 77, 3, 55–467.
Sharpe, E. (1927). 'Symposium on child-analysis', *International Journal of Psycho-Analysis*, 8, 380–384.
Sharpe, E. (1947). 'The psycho-analyst', *International Journal of Psycho-Analysis*, 28, 1–6.
Sharples, M. (1999). *How we write: writing as creative design*. London: Routledge.
Silverman, D. (2013). *Interpreting qualitative data*, fourth edition. California: Sage.
Smith, R., Parrott, W., Ozer, D. & Moniz, A. (1994). 'Subjective injustice and inferiority as predictors of hostile and depressive feelings in envy', *Personality and Social Psychology Bulletin*, 20, 6, 705–711.
Sperling, S. (1953). 'On the psychodynamics of teasing', *Journal of the American Psychoanalytic Association*, 1, 458–483.
Speziale-Bagliacca, R. (2008). 'Reverie and metaphor: a particular way to investigate the unconscious', *American Journal of Psychoanalysis*, 68, 350–359.
Spillius, E. (1996a). *Melanie Klein today: developments in theory and practice*, vol. 2: *Mainly practice*. London: Routledge.
Spillius, E. (1996b). *Melanie Klein Today. Developments in theory and practice*, vol. 1: *Mainly theory*. London: Routledge.
Spillius, E. & O'Shaughnessy, E. (2012). *Projective identification: the fate of a concept*. East Sussex: Routledge.
Srivastava, P. & Hopewood, N. (2009). 'A practical iterative framework for qualitative data analysis', *International Journal of Qualitative Methods*, 8, 1, 76–84.
Stein, S. (2001). 'Legitimising TV journalism in 60 minutes: the ramifications of subordinating the visual to the primacy of the word', *Critical Studies in Mass Communication*, 18, 3, 249–269.
Stepansky, P. (2009). *Psychoanalysis at the margins*. New York: Other Press.
Stern, A. (1948). 'Transference in borderline neuroses', *Psychoanalytic Quarterly*, 17, 527–528.
Stern, D. (1985). *The interpersonal world of the infant*. New York: Basic Books.
Sternberg, J. (2005). *Infant observation at the heart of training*. London: Karnac.
Stolorow, R. (2003). 'On the impossibility of immaculate perception – there is no relationship without interpretation, and there is no interpretation without relationship', *Progressive Self Psychology*, 19, 217–223.
Stolorow, R. & Atwood, G. (1994). 'The myth of the isolated mind', *Progressive Self Psychology*, 10, 233–250.
Stolorow, R., Atwood, G. & Orange, D. (2002). *Worlds of experience: interweaving philosophical and clinical dimensions in psychoanalysis*. New York: Basic Books.
Strachey, J. (1934). 'The nature of the therapeutic action of psycho-analysis', *International Journal of Psycho-Analysis*, 15, 127–159.
Strømme, H., Gullestad, E., Stanicke, E. & Killingmo, B. (2010). 'A widening scope on therapist development: designing a research interview informed by psychoanalysis', *Qualitative Research in Psychology*, 7, 3, 214–232.
Sullivan, H. (1954). 'Psychiatry', *Psychoanalytic Review*, 41, 66–92.

Swackhamer, G. (1937). 'Imago', *Psychoanalytic Review*, 24b, 191–202.

Tauber, E. (1949). 'Eidelberg, L. Take off your mask [New York: International Universities Press, 1948. 230 pp. $3.25]', *Psychoanalytic Review*, 36, 324–325.

Taylor, D. (2009). 'Consenting to be robbed so as not to be murdered', *Psychoanalytic Psychotherapy*, 23, 263–275.

Thorne, S. (2000). 'Data analysis in qualitative research', *Evidence Based Nursing*, 3, 68–70.

Tonnesmann, M. (1989). *About children and children-no-longer: Paula Heimann, collected papers 1942–80*. London: Routledge.

Touroni, E. & Coyle, A. (2002). 'Decision-making in planned lesbian parenting: an interpretative phenomenological analysis', *Journal of Community & Applied Social Psychology*, 12, 3, 194–209.

Tower, L. (1956). 'Countertransference', *Journal of the American Psychoanalytical Association*, 4, 224–255.

Trevarthen, C. & Aitken, K. (2001). 'Infant intersubjectivity: research, theory, and clinical applications', *Journal of Child and Adolescent Psychiatry*, 42, 1, 3–48.

Ungar, V. & de Ahumada, L. (2001). 'Supervision: a container-contained approach', *International Journal of Psycho-Analysis*, 82, 71–81.

Urwin, C. & Sternberg, J. (2012). *Infant observation and research*. London: Routledge.

Vaillant, G. (1977). *Adaptation to life*. Boston: Little, Brown.

Vendler, H. (2000). *Seamus Heaney*. Cambridge, MA: Harvard University Press.

Waddell, M. (1984). 'The long weekend', *Free Associations*, 1A, 72–84.

Waddell, M. (2000). *Inside lives*. London: Gerald Duckworth & Co.

Waddell, M. (2006). 'Infant observation in Britain: the Tavistock approach', *International Journal of Psycho-Analysis*, 87, 1103–1120.

Wallerstein, J. & Kelly, J. (1976). 'The effects of parental divorce: experiences of the child in later latency', *American Journal of Orthopsychiatry*, 46, 2, 256–269.

Weir, H. (1996). 'Analytic reverie and poetic reverie: a comparison', *Free Associations*, 6, 315–333.

Weiss, J. (1992). 'The role of interpretation', *Psychoanalytic Inquiry*, 12, 296–313.

Wengraf, T. (2001). *Qualitative research interviewing: biographic narrative and semi-structured methods*. London: Sage.

Wertz, F. (1986). 'Common methodological fundamentals of the analytic procedures in phenomenological and psychoanalytic research', *Psychoanalysis and Contemporary Thought*, 9, 563–603.

Whitehouse-Hart, J. (2012). 'Surrendering to the dream: an account of the unconscious dynamics of a research relationship', *Journal of Research Practice*, 8, 2, article M5, accessed from http://jrp.icaap.org/ on 16 December 2014.

Willis, P. & Trondman, M. (2000). 'Manifesto for ethnography', *Ethnography*, 1, 5, 5–16.

Winnicott, D. (1949). 'Hate in the counter-transference', *International Journal of Psycho-Analysis*, 30, 69–74.

Winnicott, D. (1956). 'On transference', *International Journal of Psycho-Analysis*, 37, 386–388.

Winnicott, D. (1958). 'The capacity to be alone', *International Journal of Psycho-Analysis*, 39, 416–420.

Winnicott, D. (1963). 'Communicating and not communicating leading to a study of certain opposites', reprinted in: *The maturational process and the facilitating environment: studies in the theory of emotional development*. New York: International Universities Press, 1965, 179–192.

Winnicott, D. (1965a). *The maturational processes and the facilitating environment: studies in the theory of emotional development*. The International Psycho-Analytic Library, 64. London: The Hogarth Press and the Institute of Psycho-Analysis, 1–276.

Winnicott, D. (1965b). 'A clinical study of the effect of a failure of the average expectable environment on a child's mental functioning', *International Journal of Psycho-Analysis*, 46, 81–87.

Winnicott, D. (1968). 'Playing: its theoretical status in the clinical situation', *International Journal of Psycho-Analysis*, 49, 591–599.

Winnicott, D. (1969). 'The use of an object', *International Journal of Psycho-Analysis*, 711–716.

Winnicott, D. (1971). *Playing and reality*. London: Tavistock Publication.

INDEX

Note: Appendices, figures, and text boxes are indicated by the suffixes "app", "fig", and "box" respectively. Endnotes are indicated by the suffix "n" plus the footnote number e.g. "71n1". Case studies are filed under the pseudonym and subject matter.